The Male Nurse: Addressing the myths of maleness in nursing

The Male Nurse: Addressing the myths of maleness in nursing

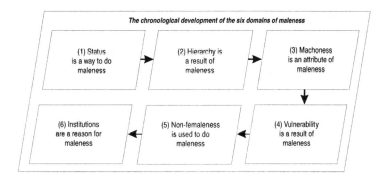

The chronological development of the six domains of maleness

(1) Status is a way to do maleness → (2) Hierarchy is a result of maleness → (3) Machoness is an attribute of maleness ↓ (6) Institutions are a reason for maleness ← (5) Non-femaleness is used to do maleness ← (4) Vulnerability is a result of maleness

Dean-David Holyoake

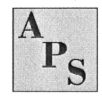

APS Publishing
The Old School, Tollard Royal, Salisbury, Wiltshire, SP5 5PW
www.apspublishing.co.uk

British Library Cataloguing in Publication Data
A catalogue record for this book is available from the British Library

© APS Publishing 2001
ISBN 1 9038770 1 6

Printed in the UK by Selwood Printing Limited, Burgess Hill

Contents

Acknowledgements

The research that supported this book needed wise and calculated insight. For this, I would like to acknowledge Bill Jessen at the University of Central England. In addition, I acknowledge Chris Brainnigan and Martin Pursey for their argumentative approach to my work. I acknowledge the nurses who trusted me enough to let me into their world and my publisher, Valery Marston, who gave instruction, support and guidance.

Introduction

Maleness is a way to do nursing

'I would not be doing justice to girls if I were to imply that they accepted all their enculturation without a struggle

(Germaine Greer, 1971: p78)

'The term Maleness is something that all of the nurses assume means 'doing manly things' ; It's something that makes the men different to the women'

(Musings from Case Study 1, Field Journal; Day 5)

This book is about the lives of male nurses who work in psychiatric nursing culture at the turn of the twentieth century. It is a book that suggests the world of the male nurse is weird, wonderful and routinely assigned, not by biology of sex, but by patriarchy and masculinity. These powerful political, ideological and cultural structures comprise of, and dictate, a discourse maintained by stereotypic gender representations. These representations go some way to produce the characteristics of psychiatric nursing culture and individual *identity* for all nurses. Male nurses are perceived to harbour natural traits that make them both suited (dealing with aggressive patients, being more caring than the average man and, perhaps, more in touch with their feminine side) and, in some ways, alien to nursing (being as sensitive as female nurses, etc). These perceptions, be they from nurses themselves or the general public, usually revolve around cultural myths regarding females being more emotional and males being more aggressive, and the like. That there is, somehow, a 'naturalness' about these identity traits that can be accounted for biologically and as peculiar to particular personalities. This type of biological individualising of gender representation often neglects to appreciate the impact cultural ideology has on the formation of nurse identity.

The perception that gender identity is not a natural and essentialist phenomenon, but a socially derived set of categories, dependent on cultural knowledge, is central to social constructionist theory. In its more extreme form, this theory might suggest that there is also no agency, freewill, or representation of typical masculine traits without cultural knowledge; a cultural knowledge that, for psychiatric nurses, is full to the brim with old traditions and new practices that cannot be divorced from specific gender representations. This book uses research taken from extensive fieldwork conducted by the author to suggest that 'maleness as a way to do nursing' is a position, from which all male nurses are judged and required to perform as the privileged sex.

Are all males the same; are men and women different?

The concept that the word 'masculinity' can be replaced by 'masculinit(ies)', a plural noted by Connell (1987), highlights an important issue in contemporary gender studies. It demonstrates the fragmented and contextual nature of modern identity (Hall and du Gay, 1996), a seemingly troublesome precept that conflicts with the traditional notions held about gender and sex types. These traditional notions focus on *difference* in attitudes and behaviours of male and females (in this case, male and female nurses) that are a direct result of their biological sex type. In this traditional view, sex type informs and is responsible for all gender-related differences.

As an eager researcher, the author spent three years using case study methodology to observe, interview and learn from nurses in three separate psychiatric nursing cultures, in an attempt to categorise all these traditional and expected sex type differences between male and female nurses. Yet, it became apparent during the fieldwork that the idea of charting and demonstrating this *difference* was not so novel, fresh or forthcoming. It reflected the general assumption in gender studies that an understanding of difference could, somehow, prove useful; it made the author ponder how useful it was for nursing practice. As the analysis of data and fieldwork progressed, it became even more apparent to the author that the study of *difference* seemed to be hiding other, deeper and missing possibilities, possibilities that could include examining what it meant for male nurses to be considered 'macho', 'power mad', or 'one of the lads'. This led to an exploration of issues relating to the implications of cultural knowledge, a knowledge that is related to powerful ideologies rather than biological trait differences.

Therefore, this book draws upon issues to do with socially constructed signs and symbols instead of naturally occurring biological sex differences. It attempts to remove itself from concepts of gender difference to those related to cultural representations and cultural meaning; issues relating to the symbolism of everyday events in psychiatric nursing practice and the reiteration of signs that go to ensure male nurses share a common culture and identity. By concentrating on the way nurses shaped their identities within inpatient nursing culture, this book offers a plausible account based upon fieldwork conducted over a period of three years. During this time, the author completed three case studies of cultures unknown to him, and conducted numerous ethnographic interviews in order to develop 'folk terms' and 'included terms' related to the signs associated with male mental health nurses.

This collection of data related to male nurses, or Maleness (males who are nurses), enabled the author to look at psychiatric nursing culture in terms of a closed system of symbols in context, i.e., as a framework of codes and signs that have contextual meaning. This approach allowed for an examination of gender issues in nursing as social constructions rather than just biological differences. This is not to ignore completely the biological differences between male and female nurses. Rather, it is to see the *influence* of biological differences and, indeed, sexuality itself, as cornerstones to the development of identity that might be partly constructed over time, through types of 'cultural layering'.

It is with this layering of cultural knowledge that the author attempted to explore how particular masculine identities had social and cultural 'meaning', how some personas are more sought after or marginalised, as having both cultural value and use, and how particular cultures consumed and then reproduced particular signs as being representative of appropriate masculine identity. It is on the friction generated, as male nurses are subjected to performing particular masquerades, that this book focusses. In particular, it centres on the relationship and conflict between individual *identity* and nursing *cultural knowledge*.

A brief outline of some of the methodological processes employed and deployed by the author during his fieldwork is given only as a guide. It was never his intention to write a book about research issues. Having said that, *Chapter 12, How to explore gender issues in psychiatric nursing culture,* is provided at the end of the book so that certain terms and research processes can be clarified in more detail. The primary objective of this book is to raise the profile of gender issues in nursing culture and provide the reader with a contemporary post-structural analysis that reflects nursing culture at the beginning of a new century.

Chapter 1
Gender issues in nursing

'In everyday life we take for granted that there are two and only two sexes'.

(Garfinkel, 1967).

Introduction

Our thoughts about gender and its relationship to nursing culture do not exist as a formalised, or co-ordinated systematic canon of theory. The perception that nursing practice would benefit from an expanded awareness and understanding of gender-related matters is seen as having little relevance to the provision of direct patient care. Yet, it might be argued that the nature of masculinity in nursing culture, although uncertain in terms of its impact, would appear far reaching, because gender constructs affect every nurse to varying degrees at different times.

The purpose of this book is to focus on the congruence of perceptions about this impact of masculinit(ies) in psychiatric nursing culture, and put forward ideas about how male nursing identity is constituted and subjected by cultural nursing knowledge. To achieve this, the book is guided by the following two aims:

1. Describe the cultural conditions and the context relating to the practice of male nurses; and

2. Identify the most prominent ideas of gender and their relationship to issues of masculinit(ies) for male nurses. (Note: The term 'masculinit(ies)' denotes the theoretical use as developed by Connell, (1987). At all other times 'masculinity' will be used).

This book focusses on the more defined concept of *masculinities* and male nurses as opposed to exploring *differences* between male and female nurses.

1

The topic of gender and cultural studies is multi-faceted and, theoretically, large. These two subjects have been approached from many varied perspectives of which some are more dominant; in particular, the feminist movement and anthropology, respectively. This plethora of empirical and phenomenological deduced and induced theory makes up the bulk of what we believe to be 'true' about gender, culture, and identity. However, within this diverse grouping, there is more disagreement than agreement at the philosophical and theoretical level, as to how gender should be explained (Davies, 1995), categorised (Buchbinder, 1998; Connell, 1987), and researched (Crowe, 1998). In summary, there are many opinions and specific research, but no general consensus. Therefore, the two overall aims of this and the following chapter are:

1. To introduce the relevant literature about theories of gender related to the ideas put forward in this book; and

2. To demonstrate how the concepts of masculinity and culture (as directly related to the focal data collected during the fieldwork) can provide the foundation for theoretical interpretation and discussion.

Gender: The study of difference

As noted by Walsh (1977), 'it is generally accepted that the study of sex *differences* and gender has a long social history'. The promotion of sex differences has had many objectives. In particular, early scientific studies on the subject sought to prove that women and the poor occupy their subordinate roles by the 'harsh dictates of nature' (Gould, 1981). *Difference* and *identity*, therefore, are the cornerstones, the underlying threads on which the fabric of gender and identity studies is woven. Evidence of the proliferation of research on gender can be seen in Matlin's book (1996), 'The Psychology of Women', which has 2,343 citations, 1167 of which have been published since 1990 (Walsh, 1997); an article a day for half a decade.

Difference is important to the gender debate because, on the one hand, the assumption that biological difference—and, therefore, biological determinism—can account for sex role attributes of men and women, competes against a difference that can also be thought of as a social construction ('doing gender' rather than sex), which is aggressively maintained by those who have social advantage, **men**.

It appears that, irrespective of one's theoretical position (sex role *vs* social constructionist), gender research has typically been seen to have kept women in a subordinate position. According to the *Boston Medical and Surgical Journal* (1896) 'women could not become doctors because of the strain of constant house calls', yet they hailed the work of nurses who regularly went out into the slums (Walsh, 1997). The publication of Maccoby and Jacklin's 'Psychology of Sex Differences' (1974) marked a major breakthrough in research on gender differences, as the two authors synthesised more than 2000 studies and concluded that gender differences had been demonstrated to exist **only** in aggression, spatial, verbal and mathematical aptitude. This was welcome news to the growing feminist movements at the time. According to Eagly (1995), feminist critiques into gender difference were fired by the expectation that findings demonstrating that women were **not** different from men would open up new opportunities for women. But difference is ingrained in every nook and cranny, in every institution in our culture, particularly that which seeks to protect the ideological status quo: patriarchy and masculinity.

According to Walsh (1997), the media is more interested in difference than similarity. This is reflected in the post-structural work of Baudrillard (1994) and his theory that all reality is self-referential due to our fascination with the 'image'. As noted by Gorman (1992), the cover of Time, for example, asked 'Why are men and women different?' while Newsweek, as noted by Shapiro (1990), focussed on 'Guns and Dolls'. The wish to consolidate similarities, as a starting point, seems to be overlooked when compared to the search for difference. In the recent and popular work of Moir and Moir (1999), there is a strong argument that there are gender differences between the two sexes, which should be acknowledged despite the claim by much mainstream feminism that difference is a social and political construction.

As noted by the influential gender theorist Unger (1992), despite the large number of theoretical papers arguing that the study of sex differences is not a relevant feminist concern, 'there has been little change in research practices' even in journals specifically dedicated to the study of women (Fine and Gordon, 1989; Lott, 1990), the study of positivism (Unger, 1989), psychological trends (Mednick, 1989) and traditional gender questions, including sex role theory (Kitzinger, 1987; Unger and Crawford, 1992). This traditionalism with the reliance on 'difference' is the typical assumption (usually based on the sex role *identities*) held up as proof of difference. The nature of research itself helps to promote difference, as in the work of Bem (1974) in her development of the androgyny theory. In the majority of this type of theory and research, there is a consistency in the historical period to which it belongs. One only has to note that work conducted during the 1970s and early 1980s will more than likely share this fascination with difference, or, by arguing against difference, draw attention to the fact that it is a common held assumption.

So what are the differences studied by gender researchers? The interest in female and male stereotypic behaviours, occupations, personality traits and so on during the 1970s came as a response to the first wave of Anglo-American feminism. For men in nursing, this attempt to 'level the playing field' had little effect. The low number of men in general nursing (approximately 10–12%: Royal College of Nursing, 1985) suggests that nursing was still considered a female occupation and is still so today. Further, it is an occupation that requires the sensitive, caring and nurturing skills that are so often stereotyped as 'naturally' belonging to the female nurse. According to Pontin (1988), the recruitment and study of men has been 'ignored for far too long'. Others share this anger. Studies related to nursing gender issues have tended to confirm the notions prevalent in the wider society (Holyoake, 1999; Davies, 1995). These assumptions being that nursing is essentially expressive in its nature and, therefore, the prerogative of women with all that this entails (Hesselbart, 1977). Some studies focussing on difference include the early work of Hoffman (1970), who found that, when compared with the wider population at large, nurses scored below average for personality traits, such as dominance, change, aggression, and autonomy. This curious suggestion now finds itself out of date, with the advent of political correctness (PC) and the growing inference that it is the individual not the role that determines the degree of the trait.

For example, Burns (1977) researched the disparity of perception in the qualities of the sexes in nursing. The main themes postulated were that women regarded men as more 'traditionally' agentic and male nurses regarded men in nursing as [politely] expressive. Overall, men view the women in nursing, as particularly emotionally labile and 'traditionally' feminine. Other key studies by Gumley *et al* (1979) and Brown and Stones (1972) have investigated the values and attitudes of men in nursing, and a similar picture emerges. Men are thought to be more aggressive and dominant, as opposed to the emotional and caring female. Similarly, studies by Lynn *et al* (1975) and Lemkau (1984) emphasise that male nurses seem to stand alone in personal qualities and make up; i.e., they differ from non-nurse males because they possess feminine characteristic that render them able to nurse. Thus, the sex difference perspective is one dominating society and nursing to such a degree that it seems to confuse the identification of *who can* and *what can* be attributed to a' good' nurse. This is an important point, because it forms part of the starting position for this book, which argues that our fascination with difference is a smoke screen for 'myths' that may appear natural or individualistic, but is, in fact, a product of a social structure: cultural knowledge.

Having acknowledged these trait differences, the question still remains as to why male nurses occupy the majority of managerial positions in nursing? Why are males over-represented, not just in management positions, but also at all levels of senior nursing hierarchy (Ratcliffe, 1996)? Most surveys and studies consistently show that, whereas men make up about 10% of the nursing work force, they make up around 35% of managerial grades (Dingwall, 1972; Austin, 1977; Nuttall, 1983; Jolley, 1989; Robinson, 1992). The usual functionalist analysis of econometric theories tend to be discourse-blind, arguing that nurses make both linear and lateral career moves and that male nurses make quicker climbs up the managerial ladder due to women's child care responsibilities. Once again, the issue becomes one of difference, as opposed to acknowledging the possibility of larger discourses of Maleness that may constitute nursing culture. The perception is that nursing has an essentially female character, and Rutty (1998) has noted that a number of authors see the nursing role as the work of wives and mothers and this includes the physical and emotional work of caring (James, 1992; Smith, 1993).

The sex differences approach is based on the theory that the main social differences between males and females are caused by, and are reflections of, biological differences. Thus, in this view 'biology is destiny'. The work of early theorists, such as Bowlby (1969; 1973; 1979), Parsons (1951) and even Freud (1995) reflect something of the 'naturalness' of sex differences. Hence, the notion of masculine and feminine characteristics being viewed as natural take on a special significance within nursing. Even in more contemporary literature being naturally feminine or masculine continues to be one of the major issues. Pontin (1988) suggests that, while men in nursing may have taken on board, or previously possessed, feminine characteristics, there still remain masculine aspects to their personalities that 'differentiate them from female nurses'. The 'good' nurse is stereotyped as attractive, compliant and female (Keddy *et al*, 1986). The good male nurse is someone who is aware of political correctness (Hollway and Jefferson, 1996), i.e., not so masculine as to warrant special feminine characteristics.

Even though the sex (biology)/gender (culture) distinction has been useful in stimulating research, it has come under increasing criticism. The main direction of this criticism is that the body itself, including its sexuality, is subject to social and personal definition and evaluation. As noted by O'Donnell (1997), Scott and Morgan (1993) have made one of the clearest rejections of the sex/gender differences model. They make the point that the body and biology, in general, are not fixed 'givens', but are subject to historical construction. Likewise, the work of Connell (1987) criticises the 'additive' approach associated with sex difference functionalism. Additives are culturally elaborated distinctions between the sexes, built upon the certain differences established by biology. In this respect, the ideology of masculinity can be viewed as an additive. This is an important consideration regarding this book, because masculinity can be viewed as either a label for actual biological distinctions, or as a label for socially constructed gender traits.

It is possible to summarise the main features discussed so far:

- The study of gender is multi-complex and open to varied and wide interpretation
- The study of gender issues in nursing has tended to be considered of little relevance to the profession
- Study of gender in nursing has tended to promote the notion of 'difference' between the sexes
- The typical view of nursing centres upon it being considered a female occupation, and this requires the 'naturally' caring and sensitive approach usually associated with femininity
- Male nurses are generally thought to be more caring and sensitive than the majority of males in the general population. However, they are second class in the 'naturally' occurring 'sex type traits', such as caring, when compared to their female counterparts
- Modern nursing is founded on a principle of individual uniqueness, i.e., it is the personality of the individual that makes the 'difference' within the confines of their gender. This theoretical position finds itself in conflict with traditional stereotype and trait theory.

Power

This section relates to two important core topics: identity (the self) and power. These two concepts are important themes explored during this book. The main concern of this section is to provide an outline of a number of significant post-structural terms and their implication for this book. First, the notion of Foucault's *subjectivization* and *the self*; and second, the issue of *knowledge* and *power*. This later work of Foucault on the effects of discourse on the subject was incomplete at the time of his death (1984).

It is assumed that the identity expressed by male nurses is formed within the culture they practice. A survey of the literature suggests three overlapping, but clearly distinguishable uses of the concept of identity within sociology: (i) self-identity, (ii) social identity, and (iii) collective identity. As noted by O'Donnell (1997), the first usage of identity emerges from the theory of the self as developed by interactionist, George Mead (1962). In terms of agency, the self is seen as a distinctly human capacity that enables people to reflect, both on themselves and on the social world, through communication and language. This allows male nurses, as individuals, to participate in the formation of their own identity. The work of Foucault (1971; 1973; 1980) rejects this. He insists that subjectivity (personal identity) is 'constituted' by social forces rather than by individuals themselves. The notion of subjectivization will be re-visited shortly.

So what about power? Much has been written on the issue of power relations between the sexes. Some of it is useful; some of it encourages the continuance of stereotypes. The following references are those considered to have been most influential to the assumptions held by nurses.

Perhaps the most regularly presented definition of power is that of Weber (1947): 'Power is the probability that one actor within a relationship will be in a position to carry out his own will despite resistance, regardless of the basis on which that probability rests'. This definition has been built on by Wrong (1979) and Lukes (1974) who suggest that power not only lies in action, but also in not acting and delegating. Authority may be considered to be the legitimate capacity to exercise power and, in nursing, is derived from the situation, expert knowledge, and the management structure (Batey and Lewis, 1982).

Related to this authority, as noted by Bowman and Thompson (1995), it is not unusual for doctors and nurses to deny that there is anything intrinsically wrong with the traditional male/female roles, as played within the traditional family; roles that have been in the health arena since Victorian times (Game and Pringle, 1983). The interest in personal power and identity seems to have taken shape, and arisen specifically, in the paradigm of behavioural psychology and, more recently, out of neo Freudian work on female psychosexual development (Fliegal, 1986). Indeed, the growing concern about individual power has been viewed as sign of progress, and is reflected in the number of specialised journals on gender (USA) that have appeared since the mid 1970s, including *Sex Roles, Psychology of Women Quarterly, Gender and Society*, and *Feminism and Psychology*. However, these journals continue to promote a sex role paradigm of enquiry about achievement for males.

It has long been accepted that high achievement and the suppression of emotion are the keystones of masculine identity (Pleck and Sawyer, 1974; Hite, 1987; 1994; Thomas, 1993). The male nurse is apparently atypical to this concept as highlighted by the studies cited at the beginning of this chapter. According to Lemkau (1984), consistent with their low status and numbers, 'occupational atypical men have attracted little research attention'. The movement of men into female-dominated domains may have an especially salutary effect with regard to enhancing the perceived prestige, power, and desirability of career choices (Touhey, 1974). Over 25 years ago, as noted by Lynn *et al* (1975), the effort to recruit males for female occupations had been performed 'in an attempt to upgrade the profession'. Increasing the number of males in the nursing profession would provide a different role model that would liberate the *symbolic identity* away from the effeminate male nurse.

However, according to Paglia (1992), this type of sexual liberation is a modern delusion, 'We are hierarchical animals. Sweep one hierarchy away, and another will take its place'. Paglia suggests that the implications of sexual domination is inseparable from western culture, 'Western culture has a roving eye. Male sex is hunting and scanning'. Carr (1996), who argues that how society views human sexuality and sexual expression determines how we act as nurses, notes this type of sexual power. Naish (1995) argues that hierarchies of power [as intimated by Paglia (1992)] must be replaced by needs-driven strategies in the health care industry. According to Huntington (1996), in the present, patriarchal power and control of all institutions in society (including science and medicine) supports the continuation of the perception that women are a problem '...if women do not develop theory, male theory will fill the gap'.

The relationship between knowledge and power is rarely acknowledged outside of post structural circles. It is refreshing to read Henderson (1994) who explains that 'knowledge is generated through the power practices'; but what if power practices are generated through knowledge? Practices that involve upward mobility, as noted by Goffman (1959), are 'the presentation of proper performances'. The work of Hewison (1995) and Sines (1994) expand this type of 'presenting self' definition and all indicate that power is inert, that is, neither good nor bad. It is worth noting that there is no consensus about what power is, but there is a general theme that it is something 'individuals' use rather than something that uses. The relationship between knowledge and power is rarely acknowledged in nursing literature.

At least three theories have offered predictions of sex differences in power use (Molm, 1986). The first, sex-role socialisation, proposes that men and women acquire different personality characteristics, skills and attitudes that predispose men to be more likely to use power. Secondly, the structural theory argues that women appear to be poorer power users only because they have differential access to power. Third, the status characteristics and expectation states theory argues that sex is a status characteristic that carries evaluation and performance connotations. Spelman (1988) attempts to resolve the difficulty of characterising sexism, racism and classism as 'interlocking' with one another. Andersen and Collins (1992) describe gender, race and class as 'interlocking categories of experience'. This image provides a more *dynamic model* than those conveyed by *additive, multiplicative* or *geometric models*.

The difficulty is that no person can experience gender without simultaneously experiencing power and class.

As noted by Faith (1994), who cites Poster (1984), Foucault takes a broader view of social structures and institutions, examining how they shape the individual (the self) and how these institutions themselves have been constituted by discourses of power. This book puts forward this position, using the focal data from the case studies to suggest that Maleness impacts on nursing culture. As Foucault (1973) states, 'there is no individual or collective identity prior to history; yet history does not determine our identity, but rather charts it'. Identity is both socially constructed and the consequence of individual and collective choices within the parameters of regulated freedoms. Hartsock (1990) argues that subjects become obliterated or, rather, 'recreated as passive objects', a world in which passivity or refusal represent the only possible choices. This subjectivity is based on the individualising of ourselves on the basis that constraints of power attract each individual to a known and recognised identity.

Chapter 2
Boys, feminism and the signs of culture

The structure of masculinity

Buchbinder (1998) asks the questions, How do males in any culture understand what 'proper' masculine behaviours, styles and attitudes might be? and, How do they recognise themselves? He answers these questions from a post-structuralist, post-feminist and social constructionist approach. He argues that culture and its images constitute powerful mechanisms, by which ideologies covering gender appropriate attitudes reinforce and affirm. This is one step less than Baudrillard (1994), who argues (while still considering the encoding and decoding model of structuralism/post-structuralism) that consumption rather than production of the image is the driving force of the ideology of signs.

Similarly, the earlier work of Tolson (1977) attempts to interpret (from a more psychodynamic approach) what the masculine experience is. He explores the limits of masculinity and the limitations of the masculine experience, by analysing the ways restrictive definitions of gender and identity are supported by social institutions. Overwhelmingly, his analysis reveals the significance of work and the workplace in the construction of the masculine identity, and its implications for patriarchal culture.

The work of Connell (1987) also provides a working model from which the question of feminism, patriarchy, masculinity, and the nature of the male nursing role can be considered. In the words of Connell, masculinity reflects 'the experience of being up against something, of limits on freedom...' The concept of 'social' structure expresses the constraints that lie in a given form of social organisation. Masculinity is seen as a limitation of freedom for male nurses. It is not only a limit on male freedom, but also a producer of 'meaning' and models of consumption at the site of the subject, in this case, psychiatric nursing culture. This issue of freedom, as well as Connell's interactional structures, provides a model, unable to divorce itself from the sex role theories that it tries to liberate. Connell progresses the gender topic by providing an analytical model, which asks new questions about masculinity. The questions asked might include: How is masculinity constructed ? How does masculinity operate or function? Is masculinity in balance or conflict? What is the relationship of the individual to their culture? These questions highlight the main theme of Connell's work; that there is not one single masculinity, but rather, one dominant masculinity with other distinct sub masculinities. Masculinity is, therefore a plural, it is masculinit(ies).

However, due to the lack of appropriate substitutes, Connell has to rely on typical representations of behaviours that go to make up each of these masculinities. For example, the nature of gay masculinity is recognised by certain behaviours—an outcome of this study being the folk term 'acting straight'. In addition, Connell's structural model is an outlining of the main parts of gender relationships and how they work. He suggests that there are three major institutional areas to be considered: (i) Labour, (ii) Power, and (iii) Cathexis (personal relations). It is with the latter that the author used Connell's model to begin piecing together the nature of masculinities in nursing. The starting point is based on the premise that all behaviour is social. For example, to recognise sexuality (in terms of acting straight), it is necessary first to see sexuality as a collection of social representations. Although he does not expand his argument, or even acknowledge the implications of encoded and decoded symbols for how representation and identity acts on the individual, he does acknowledge that the three institutional areas are interrelated, and that the relationship between them can change. He concludes that change occurs because individuals and groups strive to make change happen.

The notion that individuals, as a cultural collective, can create change may go some way to show how Connell distrusts structuralist philosophy. He asserts that individuals have agency. He views the individual as being able to interact in a dynamic and purposeful way with others to form a self, an identity. This book proposes that Connell's model provides some useful perspectives, but questions regarding the individual, identity, and agency are under-examined, even though they are not Connell's major concern. Herein lies the conflict with this book and the end of Connell's usefulness, because the development of the ethnographic themes and discussion in this book support the opinion that there is no self outside of the discourse: that identity and subjective agency are a product of cultural knowledge. Having said that, Connell's model provides us with the notion of plural masculinities, and his ideas about gender order and gender regimes reflect the determined nature of everyday experience for nurses.

For Connell, hegemonic masculinity is the dominant form of masculinity in society as a whole. For male nurses, it is the charge nurse who has earned respect, through rolling up his sleeves, getting stuck in and sustaining the pressure, who is respected by all those working under and with him. He reflects the Humphrey Bogart, John Wayne and Tom Cruise characters, cited by Connell, as being representative of hegemonic masculinity in Western society. The subordinate masculinities that always exist in relation to hegemonic masculinity, include homosexuality (which is seen to be the opposite of what a real man is) and the incompetent geek and nerd. Subordination is linked to access to power and cultural identity.

Similarly, an essential part of Connell's model is that behaviours and attitudes, often associated with masculinity and femininity, can characterise members of either sex. Given his argument that sex/gender is socially constructed, it follows that changes in social or personal circumstances may lead to changes in gender identity. Hence, the assumption given by the early works of nurse theorists, that male nurses often seem to have feminine characteristics when compared to the male population as a whole.

Moving the argument forward, it is possible to examine the work of Martin Mac an Ghaill's, The Making of Men (1985), which studies the processes involved in the interplay between schooling, masculinities (plural—similar to those proposed in Connell's model) and sexuality. Most of the empirical material in the book is based on an ethnographic study of male students, similar to that performed with male nurses during this study. Mac an Ghaill states that his primary concern was with the question of how school processes helped shape male students. This mirrors (in part) the concern of our interest when we ask how does masculinity in nursing culture shapes identity for male nurses ? Mac an Ghaill makes full reference to other agencies of socialisation, especially family socialisation, and to the influence of structural forces, such as the labour market. He distinguishes four main types of emergent heterosexual masculinity:

(i)   The macho lads (marginalised masculinity)

(ii) The academic achievers (upwardly mobile)

(iii) New enterprises, and

(iv) The real Englishmen (middle-class).

It should be noted that the term, 'machoness', in this book was adapted in terms of the ethnographic styling.

Buchbinder (1998), Mac an Ghaill (1985), Connell (1987) and Tolson (1977) provide a foundation from which to begin an exploration of masculinity in nursing. However, there are a number of retrospective points worthy of note. Connell's main contribution, as noted by O'Donnell (1997), is to loc- ate—persuasively and in detail—masculinities and patriarchy itself within the wider concept of gender. Masculinities are aspects of a wider structure—the gender order. Possibly, without exception, every gender order in the world is, to a greater or lesser extent, patriarchal. Both Connell and Mac an Ghaill arguably provide the most complete and developed theoretical account of gender so far achieved. In addition, the psychodynamic approach of Tolson, and the interest in cultural imagery and myth presented by Buchbinder, provide us with four approaches that give an extensive and contemporary theoretical foundation.

Each theorist leans towards a social constructionist approach in his/her quest to understand the various issues of masculinity with which he/she is concerned. For this study, it is *identity*; for Tolson, it is work and family, for Mac an Ghaill, it is social pressure, and for Connell, it is a number of factors motivated by a society that categorises and is 'additive'. The question of agency of individuals is typically interactionist for Connell and a process of psychoanalytical stage development for Tolson. It seems that both Mac an Ghaill and Buchbinder argue that individuals and their freedom are constituted by discourse.

Feminism

The principle perspective in gender literature is dominated by groups of theory that are either feminist, or seemingly categorised by how anti-feminist they are. Although it is not the aim of the author to focus too much upon feminism, it is necessary to draw attention, if only briefly, to the sub-types that belong to it. Types of feminism have traditionally been categorised into four groups. These are Marxist feminism, radical feminism, liberal feminism (which are all seen as belonging to Anglo-American schools of thought) and, more recently, post-feminism (European). A brief definition of what feminism is can be drawn from an essay entitled 'What is feminism?' by Delmar (1986). Following the example of Simone de Beauvoir (1949), 'A feminist is someone who is concerned with: (i) Discrimination against women; (ii) Unsatisfied needs of women; (iii) The necessity for radical change if these needs are not met'.

In the 1970s, a number of feminists began to draw on the work of Marx to explain the oppression of women. These writers included: Sharpe (1972), Mitchell (1971) and Chodorow (1978). In short, these Marxist feminists stress the need to overthrow the capitalist economic system so that an ideological shift can occur in the consciousness of **both** sexes.

Radical feminism is not Marxist and is based on the analysis that patriarchy and masculinity rather than capitalism are the central issue to be faced by feminists. Writers, such as

Millett (1970), Firestone (1972) and Greer (1971; 1984; 1999), see the ideological reproduction of patriarchy as detrimental to women, in particular, the way females become willing collaborators in their own oppression. This is of particular relevance, because male nurses may argue that they have no choice but to represent masculinity in a certain way, in order to practice the role they are also forced to adopt.

Where both Marxist and radical feminists stress the need for structural change, liberal feminism is a reformism approach. It supports the use of legal and educational change for the benefit of females in the work place and home. Today, we find ourselves in a period known as post-feminism. It signifies a shift in feminist theory. Such an approach uses post-structural and postmodern philosophy to progress towards gender *equality* and an understanding of gender *identity*. It is useful to consider some of the issues at the core of post-feminism because they reflect the concerns of this book.

Post-feminism draws attention to the linguistic differentiation associated in English with the two adjectives for the terms woman and man. One adjective derivation—feminine and masculine—is used by feminists to refer to social, cultural, and psychic constructions. The distinction, as noted by Phoca and Wright (1999), can be broadly understood as 'an ideological one'. Five hundred years of humanism has supported the view that individuals, regardless of sex, can be free autonomous, free-thinking beings (Crowe, 1998).

The humanist tradition puts forward the view that human self-improvement is unlimited and, although some post-feminists would disagree, most post-feminist theory is based on anti-humanist philosophy, which tends to emphasise the social, economic, and psychological structures that determine and limit the ways in which an individual can act. The story of sexuality, the Oedipus complex, penis envy, the mother's body, and object relations theory, to name just a few, can all be analysed as being limiting factors, trapped within the confines of discourse. They are considered elites of knowledge, yet can be critiqued, using postmodern and post-feminist analysis, as being unstable views of reality. The work of Irigaray (1992), Paglia (1992), Pateman (1988),

Kristeva (1982), and Mitchell (1971) can all be referenced as making a considerable contribution to the progression of post-feminist issues, by emphasising the contained nature of semiotics, language, and culture.

The importance of *'difference'*, as concluded from mainstream sex role/trait gender theory, makes real the identity, cultural reality, individual power, and the seemingly inert nature of language, as a collection of issues that are, in the words of Connell (1987), 'additives'. That is, they are packaged topics that can be thought of as being somehow additional or related to gender.

Cultural meaning and language

It is important to consider gender representation as a key concept in the aim of this book, to understand the 'meaning' of masculinity for nurses in context, and how cultural meaning (signs) about masculinity and Maleness impact on male nurses and nursing culture. Representation, as defined by Hall (1997), is one of the central practices that produces culture meaning and a key 'moment' in, what has been called, the 'circuit of culture' (du Gay, 1997). The idea that culture can be considered a circuit rather than an historical linear evolution is an idea that has been progressed by post-structural and postmodern thinkers during the past thirty years. It is argued that culture is about shared 'meanings', without shared meanings there is no culture. Language is the privileged medium in which we make sense of things, in which meaning is produced and exchanged. Meanings can only be shared through our common access to language. Meaning is constructed in and through language (constructionist) rather than being a simple reflection of meaning that already exists (reflective), or as an expression of what a person wants to say (intentional). The study of meaning (using a structural and post-structural model) makes use of the semiotic approach greatly influenced by Saussure (1959) and then developed by Barthes (1996), and the discursive approach associated with Foucault (1980). This simplified order will now be examined.

Linguistics is the study of language. The term 'semiotics' is used to refer to all signs not just language. The work of Spradley (1979) and his DRS is firmly rooted to the principles of Saussure, who said that language is a closed system with no universally fixed concepts. The whole of language is a system of syntagmatic and paradigmatic, negative relations of *difference*. What this means is that signs are assigned meaning, which are not naturally fixed, and that we understand what they 'mean' because they are *different* from all other signs. The words in this sentence have meaning because they individually signify something different. Yet, they are all words, assigned symbols/signs that have shared meaning—words make sentences. Neither things in themselves, nor the individual users of language can fix meaning in language. Things do not just mean: we construct meaning, using representational systems—concepts and signs (Hall, 1997).

Both sounds (language) and material objects can function as signs. Signs are made up of two parts: the signifier and the signified. The signifier is the form (word, behaviour, object) that triggers the mental concepts—the signified. Signifiers have to be organised into systems of *'difference'* (contrast sets) for them to operate, thus language has a distinctive way of organising the world into concepts and categories (taxonomies). What is true of sounds is true of ideas. Ready made ideas do not exist before words. The functionalist assumption that social phenomena must be explained by finding their hidden utilitarian functions is not useful in this way. Some important forms of behaviour have no literal utility at all. Their significance is revealed only when they are related negatively to other social phenomena at a deeper level of analysis. They are what Barthes (1996) terms **Myths**. These will be discussed in the following section.

The issue of individual essences and agency is an important consideration. All the nurse informants, who participated in the study, argued that they have complete autonomy as individuals. In addition, the cultural myths indicate that the cultural meaning reinforces the notion of the individual practitioner. However, if we agree that there is no cultural meaning without language, and that language, apart from being present before we are born, is the medium that we use to think, we can see that all individuals are part of a system: a system in which the conventions that tie the signifier to the signified is arbitrary; that is, there are no fixed universal concepts. 'Human societies, like individuals, never create absolutely; all they can do is create certain combinations' (Strauss 1963a).

The study of culture within the post-structuralist theory developed from Saussure's original encoding/decoding linguistics model. In particular, it emphasises the ability to analyse the sign into its two component parts: the signifier and the signified. The development of post-structuralism occurred as theorists applied this principle to signs that were not spoken, i.e., to the observations and symbols occurring when people interact. The emphasis is placed upon, what Barthes (1996) terms, the 'connotation' of a sign (here meaning: of maleness as represented by male nurses) and the larger structures, called discourse by Foucault (1980).

Semiotics, myths and discourse

The underlying argument behind the semiotic approach is that, since all cultural objects convey meaning and all cultural practices depend on meaning, they must make use of signs and, in so far as they do, they must work as language works, and be amenable to an analysis that, basically, makes use of Saussure's linguistic concepts of the sign (signifier + signified = sign) (Hall, 1997). The work of Barthes (1996) uses Saussure's model and applies it to cultural themes, concepts, and meanings. Barthes uses the terms *denotation* and *connotation* to refer to cultural signifiers of cultural themes. Denotation refers to the basic and simple meaning, e.g., that a nurse is making a bed. Connotation refers to the more complex level, which needs de-coding: that it is a nurses' job to make beds, to make them feel useful, refute self-care models of practice, and reinforce the maternal home roles that patients are accustomed to. All cultural signs will have both denotation and connotation to be a complete sign. An understanding of both is necessary to analyse the realms of social ideology, conceptual frameworks, and value systems of a culture.

Barthes model also proposes the notion of the 'Myth'. For a proper semiotic analysis one must be able to outline precisely the different steps by which this broader meaning has been produced, as with the taxonomic and domain analysis of this study. In Myth, representation takes place through two separate, but linked processes. For example, in the first place the signifiers and the signifieds unite to form a sign with a simple denoted message, a nurse talking to a patient in the day room. At the second stage, this completed message is linked to a second set of signifieds—a broader ideological theme about caring and listening to patients, the use of good interpersonal skills, and the therapeutic value of interaction. This second level of signification is the level of the myth. An example is given in *Figure 2.1*.

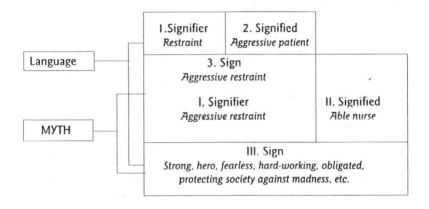

Figure 2.1: MYTH: Restraining an aggressive patient (adapted from source: Barthes, 1996, p114)

So, what good is this type of cultural analysis? How useful is the idea of the myth for analysing culture? To answer these questions, we must first remind ourselves of the definition of culture. Within the anthropological perspective, it is defined 'as a way of life' [about which 'differences' can be studied] (binary oppositions and difference give signs their meaning).

For this ethnographic research, the definition is extended from this 'way of life' position to include a focus on the *production and exchange of 'meaning'*. Therefore, returning to the two questions, it can be argued that the work of Barthes has provided a systematic and scientific method of analysing the everyday occurrences in nursing culture. Indeed, the work of Spradley's (1979) DRS concerns itself with a more intricate examination of the denotation, due to his insistence on building emic taxonomies of folk terms that do not only indicate the sign and, therefore, the possible semantic relationship between all signs. The DRS provides a research sequence that, as a model, searches the signifieds by linking all the possible signifiers.

Although Spradley is more concerned with the non-translation of ethnography, the usefulness of Barthes, and of Foucault, provides this study with the tools to explore the connotations of the ethnographic taxonomies. The search for the broader cultural themes was operationalised using Barthes' model, the cultural theme being about the shared knowledge (regarding male nurses) and the representation of maleness. In practice, this meant understanding how nurses use language to say something meaningful about, or to represent the world meaningfully to other people. Thus, the essential part of the process, by which 'meaning' is produced, consumed, and exchanged between members of a nursing team, can be thought of as shared *knowledge*. This *knowledge* uses mental representations (cognitive maps) to make use of the similarity and contrast principles (Spradley, 1979) between concepts to distinguish them from one another. Concepts are organised into relationships with each other and 'meaning' is dependent upon the relationship (semantic) between them.

Understanding nursing culture is to understand the shared meaning of relationships between concepts. Concepts are signs and symbols that are assigned 'meaning', which is constructed by the system of representation. Therefore, culture can be thought of as shared conceptual maps, shared language systems, and codes that govern the relationship of translation between them (Hall, 1997). Representation uses material objects, but the meaning depends not on the material quality of the sign, but on its *symbolic function*. Cultural analysis of the symbolic function can, therefore, be used as a means of decoding signs and the signification process (the process of assigning meaning to signs). Cultural analysis of this kind has also been the interest of other theorists, including Levi- Strauss (1966; 1963; 1063a), Lacan (1968), Derrida (1976), Lyotard (1979), and Baudrillard (1994).

Durkheim (1967) and especially Parsons (1951) saw culture largely in terms of its contribution to social order. The idea of 'symbolism' was noted by Durkheim, who saw symbolism as an opportunity for collectives to share emotional, as well as ideological beliefs. This search of 'mechanical solidarity' led him away from issues focussing specifically on individual identity, which he considered to be within the realms of psychology, in particular, the psychoanalytic theories of Erikson (1963) and Freud (1997). He was not at all concerned with the motives and 'meanings' individuals attach to their own actions. Likewise, Parson focussed on culture rather than individual agency in most of his theoretical analysis. Therefore, the issue of representation was a second cousin in comparison to the functional order of society, which could be thought of as a system.

What concerned Foucault was the production of knowledge (rather than just meaning) through what he called discourse (rather than just language) (Hall, 1997). His project was to analyse how human beings understand themselves in our culture, and how our knowledge about 'the social, the embodied individual, and shared meanings' comes to be produced in different periods. With its emphasis on cultural understanding and shared meanings, Foucault's project was still, to some degree, indebted to Saussure and Barthes. His major topics of interest were the concept of discourse, the issue of power and knowledge, and the question of the identity.

Discourse defines and produces the objects of our knowledge. It governs the way that a topic can be meaningfully talked about and reasoned. It influences how ideas are put into practice and used to regulate the conduct of others. Meaning and meaningful practice is constructed within discourse. Nothing that is meaningful exists outside discourse. The term 'discourse' is used to emphasise that every social configuration is meaningful. Foucault (1980) argues that since *'we can only have a knowledge of things if they have meaning, it is discourse—not the things in themselves—which produces knowledge.'* So, for example, for this book, the discourse of Maleness utilised the following ideas :

- statements about Maleness that give us a certain kind of knowledge about it, e.g., men and women are *different*, men in nursing are more feminine, men are more sexual
- the rules that pertain to certain ways of talking about these topics and exclude other ways—rules that govern what is 'sayable' or 'thinkable' about Maleness, e.g., females are better nurses because they are *naturally* more caring
- 'subjects' who in some way personify the discourse, e.g., the macho male nurse, the non 'straight acting' male nurse
- how this knowledge acquires authority, a sense of embodying the 'truth' about it, e.g., in this age of individualism, it is the individual practitioner who makes good or bad choices, not his/her sex
- the practices within institutions for dealing with subjects, e.g., the expectations placed on nurses to represent formal conduct.

Foucault became more concerned with how knowledge was put to work through discursive practices in specific institutional settings. Knowledge and power operates within, what he calls, institutional *apparatus* and its *technologies* (techniques). There is no power relation without the correlative constitution of a field of knowledge: 'what we think we know'. He places the body at the centre of the struggles between different formations of power and knowledge. The body is produced within discourse and it is the discourse, not the subjects who speak it, which produces knowledge. 'One has to dispense with the constituent subject, to get rid of the subject itself, that is to say, to arrive at an analysis which can account for the constitution of the subject within a historical framework' (Foucault, 1980). Discourse constructs *'subject positions'*.

Discourses are bearers of various historically specific positions of agency and identity for individuals. It is these subject-positions that provide the conditions for individuals to act or know in relation to particular social practices. The question of subjectivization is concerned with understanding the process by which individuals come to inhabit particular discursive subject positions, for example, male nurses. Foucault was interested in the emergence of modern forms of individuality through the growth of new bodies of knowledge and networks of power. Discourse works on the individual, subjecting the individual. Individual identity is the representations as performance based upon the citing and reiteration of discursive norms.

Summary

This chapter has emphasised that cultural and gender studies are composite and complex (at many levels) areas of research interest. If one were to perform just one search, thousands of references could be exacted from hundreds of sources, which would demonstrate that the issue is multi faceted, layered, and historical. Therefore, the quest and achievement of this chapter has been to superficially bracket contemporary theory into the specific sections of research epistemology, gender studies, masculinity, and cultural studies in order that a critical and more useful sorting of this huge cannon of work, not only identifies the boundaries of itself, but directs and provide the means by which this book can progress.

The issues highlighted in these first two chapters show that the study of difference; feminism; the structure of masculinity; cultural meaning and language; semiotics, myths and discourse; and power bring together many competing theories about what gender and culture are. The central theoretical considerations concern the everyday, commonly-held myths in psychiatric nursing culture and the formation of identity for male nurses. It can be seen that the theories associated with power, cultural meaning, language, and difference are all relevant for an interpretation of the focal data to be made.

Chapter 3
The impact of domain maleness

'As a result of the status difference, boys have higher expectations for success and evaluate their performance more favourably than do girls.

Linda L Carli (1997, p50)

'I think that nurses are nurses. There isn't a conspiracy to be any better, but to improve things generally ...

...you know, there are good male nurses and there are good female nurses.'

John (2) (Case 3 Interviews)

Status is a way to do maleness

Introducing the status domain

This chapter uses the ethnographic domain, 'Status is a way to do maleness' to emphasise that male nurses' identity and status is culturally determined; that their nursing status is a product of cultural meaning. Maleness (being a male nurse) constitutes a status identity (for good or ill) that is written on the body of every male nurse. There is no escaping its presence, for this is the symbolic body of the privileged male half whose identity is constituted for them, as they actively masquerade this body as a type of status performance, observed in the' swagger of the walk', in the difficult-to-detect symbols that 'male nurses are secretly proud of being good at restraint', or privileged membership as one of the biologically stronger 'hunters' of the tribe. The points for this chapter relate to:

1. Nursing culture ideologically promotes individual identity characteristics as primary facets of practice

2. In this way, identity and status are credited to the skilful use of self as a practitioner, manager, nurse consultancy, and the like

3. Male nurses simulate particular male masquerades in order to represent culturally constituted status identity
4. This simulation only has 'meaning' due to nursing cultural knowledge
5. The symbolic body represents identity and status order. As men, male nurses are subjected to perform maleness
6. Identity (or the representation of maleness) is, therefore, not autonomous, but determined by the subjectivization of maleness discourse
7. All subjects actively (re)produce, rather than passively produce, gender identity in nursing.

The aim of this chapter is to argue that status is an important cultural theme relating to psychiatric nursing culture, because it allows for an examination of the process known as subjectivization and, as such, demonstrates a more progressive analysis and discussion. The assumptions made by and about male nurses in psychiatric culture comprise a certain kind of knowledge. It is almost certain that the rules that prescribe certain ways of talking about these topics, and exclude others, are a result of nursing ideologies, some of which influence the male body to masquerade and perform in a number of ways. Therefore, we would expect male psychiatric nurses to have certain traits (which are not biologically determined) given the way cultural knowledge about the topic is constructed at this present time. But how does this cultural knowledge acquire authority; an authority that gives a sense of embodying the 'truth' of what constitutes status and how male nurse status should be performed in psychiatric nursing culture? And, perhaps, just as importantly, from where does this knowledge of status come?

The importance of the identity status symbol

In 1922, the sociologist, Max Weber, had this to say about status:

> 'The term 'social status' will be applied to a typically effective claim to positive or negative privilege with respect to social prestige so far as it rests on one or more of the following bases:

(a) mode of living, (b) a formal process of education which may consist in empirical or rational training and the acquisition of the corresponding modes of life, or (c) on the prestige of birth, or of an occupation.' (Weber, 1947 p428).

This quotation holds within it the broad concepts from which a large number of sociological definitions of status have been developed. Weber can be accused of imposing a universal grand narrative that emphasises the *role of the individual,* their education, their class (economics), and manner of occupation as a totality of identity. This familiar definition has survived almost one hundred years and has traditionally focussed on the dynamic and flexible nature of personal autonomy. Yet, Weber fails to provide an answer to the dilemma of why certain positions are given more prestige than others, and why some groups are able to obtain higher income, wealth, and respected identity than others. Similarly, the second dominant tradition, as advocated by Marxist approaches, emphasises the economic relation identity has to status. The debate about identity status has typically resulted in a seemingly common-sense agreement that some jobs are more important to society than others, and that these jobs require the most able people to fill them. Therefore, the domain, ' Status is a way to do maleness' also appears to be a 'natural' theme of this thesis for two reasons. First, it reflects the Weberian, Marxist and Functionalist concepts of status, all rolled up into what the informants assume is a truthful explanation of their everyday experiences. In this way, the issue of status is informant led; it has a real life importance for the nurses working in psychiatric nursing culture. Thus, the second reason why a discussion about status and its symbolism is important relates to the idea that, by its very absence, the lack of the 'status issue' would weaken any work concerned with culture.

The importance of status, as defined by traditional sociology, cannot be ignored, because most informants assume from their own experience that it is a true reflection in their everyday lives. The nurses in the case studies tell of these 'socio-traditional' meanings of status and represent it within their working environments. At the broad level, this can be heard in the comments of non-trained staff who, according to sociologists and theoretical models, would be a lower class of occupation (and, indeed, nursing *per se* would be considered lower than medicine, law and architecture) than a trained nurse and would, therefore, have to rely upon social prestige for their status recognition. Thus, the long serving nursing assistant (NA) would have status due to her or his length of service and experience, as opposed to the ability to write care plans. This was often demonstrated during the observation periods when nurses spoke about 'how good NAs were at talking with patients', yet 'they have no qualifications'. The analysis of status in terms of economic class, social prestige, and birth right, although traditional, provides only one model with which to examine gender and cultural issues in psychiatric nursing culture.

Most NAs in the case studies would not consider themselves an underclass or alienated. The use of these sociological terms to present a sense of universalism is not useful in this respect. The use of taxonomies and domains on the other hand allowed for a deeper analysis that, at times, appeared universal, but aimed to provide a more balanced appreciation of the cultural status expectations. It also allowed for an argument regarding the inversion of this traditional model of status to occur, i.e., the idea that cultural knowledge via subjectivization is responsible for the definition of what status is rather than class, race, age, and so on. In this form, the idea that individuals, via an essentialised identity, produce a status for themselves over time can be looked at in a different way. Nurses 'know the signs' and cosume in equal measure to producing status representations that nursing culture demands have 'sign value'. Therefore, consumption can be considered just as important, if not more so, in the production of nursing cultural symbols. Consumption of symbols ensures they continue in one form or another.

Searching for the symbols of identity

The taxonomic analysis and ethnographic theme analysis confirm that most nurses think status is about a personal identity, something correlated to personal characteristics of which gender is only a small consideration. The primary symbol of identity in nursing is seen to be the use of skilful nursing interventions with patients. This highlights the way that status, as a social phenomenon, is in a constant state of flux for nurses at any given time. The fieldwork is a window into this phenomenon and a way of exploring nursing culture, and how 'individual social agents' make sense of their subjective realities; a reality that they believe is 'out there', objective, and one in which they have status because they are 'hard working' and have 'earned respect'. These high status identities reflect that male nurses feel free to create any identity they want, but, in practice, they are pushed (and push themselves) towards identities that represent the perceived values of nursing culture. These representations are signs of cultural meaning.

No nurse can stand outside nursing cultural knowledge. Status is bestowed on individual nurses by their colleagues, and is represented using symbols that have cultural meaning and value. Some of the symbols are at the core of what is considered 'best practice' in psychiatric nursing culture. The representation of being 'supportive', 'being good at talking with patients', 'knowing you're stuff and 'being reliable' are symbols, cultural performances, and personal 'masquerades' that, not only represent 'valued' and, therefore, desirable nursing cultural knowledge, but are also 'constituted by it' (Buchbinder, 1998). In this way, status symbols and status representation maintains a consistency. In addition, the symbols of identity are viewed as being about personal *essences* or personality traits and essentialised as being fundamental in the provision of a highly qualified skill mix in the nursing team.

The sex of a nurse is seen to be predetermined and, therefore, the basic building block of a natural and essentialised identity. However, even though gender and sex provides two of the few constant measures of identity and status, this status cannot be said to be universal for all male nurses. Different male nurses have different types of status, irrespective of whether or not the meaning of that gender status remains constant within a given nursing culture. This is because the status systems in nursing arise in response to definite cultural meanings and desires. These are communicated through dominant nursing and maleness ideologies and would be defined by Barthes (1996), as ideological myths and by Foucault (1980), as elements of discourse. The symbols of maleness are peculiar to nursing and might be referred to by Baudrillard (1994), as simulating the myths and discourse of wider cultural knowledge. Therefore, some nursing signs are seen as useful and desirable (at present, sensitive, 1990s emotionally aware men) and some a warning (sexually oppressive, too quick to restrain, lazy).

So, what is the primary myth of psychiatric nursing culture? There is an assumption that nurses behave the way they do because they choose to (given the immediate resources available to them) and that they think autonomously, and gender plays little part in autonomous thinking. It has often been said that it is the responsibility of the individual male nurse to assert himself and to nurse in a way that is natural to him; perhaps, to be himself, to work in a way that is 'unique' to him or 'do his own thing'. The cultural theme is, therefore, that identity in relation to gender is natural and, therefore, somehow *biologically determined* and excusable (it would be inconceivable to assert that gender assignments are neither a natural, nor a perpetual identity). Informants told how they conform and, inevitably, draw on the available traits of gender, age, race, and class when they nurse, but that these concepts are a part of what makes them *'naturally unique, autonomous individuals'*. The myth is that it is these elements, which make up their sense of self (their identity) as they clamber up the status league. But these elements (thought to be pre-determined) provide only the bedrock on which 'the real' symbols of identity can be found. Nurses were eager to disclose other status symbols to support the argument that they were not, what Foucault (1980) would term, 'ideological subjects' and, what Baudrillard (1994) terms, 'consumers of simulated self referential signs' .

Each individual nurse has something that they are proud of because their peers confirm identified skills. The identity of individual nurses is historical, consistent, memorable, and sometimes based on fantasy. They are recognisable by these skills and images, which give them identity and a degree of status. This type of status is thought to be the best status afforded to a nurse because it is a recognition of his/her clinically based skills. Nurses identity is a clinical skill that has cultural meaning. There sits the primary myth, i.e., the most prominent ideology of nursing and maleness discourse. The nurse who displays the right symbols via performance at the right time for consumption sake (Baudrillard (1994) is awarded recognition for his/her performance (his/her (re)production of valued and desirable signs). Nurses identity becomes iconic as they replicate and reproduce textbook or high experience skills. They are seen to be 'naturals at nursing' as their identity gets sucked into the performance and erased from the essentialised core of personal trait characteristics, usually to the applause of 'John's good at doing objectives with the students' or 'Simon is good at doing the off duty'. The point being that, in the first place, it is the performance, (re)production, representation and Baudrillardian (1994), simulation' [in that order], which generates accolades and status-related recognition. In the same way, Connell (1987) and Mac an Ghaill (1985) would categorise particular traits, such as the 'macho lads' or the 'real English men'. Secondly, identity is seen not to be founded on a personal inner core, but consistent replication (reproduction) and the continued consumption of dominant ideological symbols within a nursing culture. This type of identity is a (re)production of previous performances and a simulation of known and 'valued' signs. It is self-referential. It refers to itself and status is awarded to the body that performs and repeats it.

The author has been told on many occasions that certain male nurses were very logical in their care planning and supervision of junior staff. When observed, it could be seen that they were relaxed, reflexive, set aims and objectives, and the like. Using these types of approaches signified the best of psychiatric nursing culture. They masqueraded the image. The ideology was pulling the strings of their performance, as they simulated in their, 'aren't I confident' manner, the classic business school approach to nursing. This simulation would not be out of place in a management degree, or service manager's handbook.

In this way, as Barthes (1996) might say, 'the myth is hidden' and Baudrillard (1994) might add, 'hides the in-authenticity of the skills against which nurses are allotted status and a sense of identity'. A nurse who can manipulate the symbols and perform in front of the correct audience will not be deprived of status identity. The emic view, as shown in the taxonomies, promotes and defends the notion that all nurses are different due to the essential inner core identity. There is a belief that authentic performance comes from a detachable individual who relates to a world 'out there', but the possibility that nursing reality is made up of simulation that is (self-referring signs) and (re)production makes such authenticity impossible, because all symbols refer to other simulated signs. Therefore, the second point, with respect to the essentialised autonomous identity, is that the nature of reality 'out there' is unstable. The symbols that circulate in psychiatric nursing culture are (re)productions, which appear natural, although they are, in fact, ideological. None are more so than as those myths concerned with gender difference.

So what is the impact of this difference? Maleness has a huge impact on the nursing culture in which it resides. Contrary to the general assumption held by the nurse informants, myths incite representations of what it is to be a male nurse, representations of different identities and, therefore, a different status for male nurses. Some of the folk terms, taken from the preliminary taxonomic analyses of *Case 2*, go to support this idea that male biological status is an identity most sort after by male nurses and, thus, representing a peculiar influence on the cultural meaning of psychiatric nursing culture; that the sex males are born determines the way male nurses should act and, thus, perform. Males should 'go out and work', 'bring in the money' and pay the mortgage' (folk terms from *Case 2*). This is legitimised as being responsible for having a job; this is a manly thing to do, irrespective of the fact that female nurses do the same. Likewise, the way male nurses gain status by being 'detached', 'avoiding', and not being responsible for bad atmospheres', 'not being boring', 'deciding what is an unequal work load', and 'being good management material' are all recognisable signs of how status *is a way to do* maleness.

More evidence includes the folk terms accredited to the semantic relationship, 'Status *is an attribute* of maleness'. Male nurses are expected to 'build careers', 'allowed to be more demanding' (sometimes the more demanding means more status), 'confident', and 'independent'. This type of status identity of male nurses is about 'putting on a front', 'remaining calm', 'doing the rough jobs' (restraining aggressive male patients—usually, big) and 'giving advice'. These are 'all ways to do status', and typify the unresolved issue that there is difference between male and female nurses. The symbols of maleness are regarded as commodities that male nurses do not necessarily produce as 'individuals' (rather they (re)produce), because there is a value placed on the consumption of maleness within nursing culture. During an interview, Steve (*Case 1*) raised the issue that nursing behaviours are learned. They are practised, tested, and then compared to those of other nurses. In the case of gender, such practice is never considered as a contributing factor about the care given by men. Remembering that, 'they [male nurses] are what they are' the *denotation* of the myth appears to be a sign/symbol that is signed, sealed, and delivered (encoded and decoded) as a fact of life that has no real practical or specific consequences. Yet, the same male informants simulate nursing skills as a sign of status, the *connotation* being that they 'know what they are doing'. Their status is assumed to be identified by their individuality, rather than to the correct or incorrect use of their performance (including the body) to (re)produce the standards expected within cultural knowledge. This includes their own sense of achievement and failure.

The identity of being a male nurse, as noted in the extract given by James and Liam, show that male nurses spend a considerable amount of time rationalising about status identity and their subjectivization:

> '...I definitely think that female patients view me differently...I think they see me more as a nurse who cheers them up...I don't think I do it intentionally, but it does happen.'

'...*I think that we make patients feel safe, by just being around them...*'

(James; Case 3 Interviews)

Making patients 'feel safe', as described by James, ensures that males in psychiatric nursing will continue to have a role, which is distinct (even though not acknowledged as being culturally influenced) from their female colleagues. The fact that all patients can be safe when there are no male staff on hand is difficult to explain. The idea that male staff cheer patients up is not only derogatory to female nurses, but also for the male nurse. Donning the clown suit seems to be a pre-requisite of identity and status for male nurses, who wear a particular type of symbolic body.

So, in summary, the primary myth: that psychiatric nurses are autonomous, freethinking individuals with an essential inner core has to be questioned. This can be done in at least three ways. First, that in order to have 'meaning' all symbols have to be constituted in nursing cultural knowledge. Therefore, a nurse (re)producing these cultural symbols is already subjectivized to the dominant ideologies and seduced by the cultural myths of essentialism and universalism. Second, that performance by subjects is about representing those symbols, which are privileged, in order to convey meaning. Nurses are not the individual authors of symbols. Third, the idea that reality is, itself, an illusive and troublesome concept, because of its 'self-referentiality' (Baudrillard, 1994), i.e., myth promotes particular masquerades, especially in the context of gender issues.

The symbolic body

The representations, as listed in the taxonomies, go to support the argument that both sexes find themselves having to represent, in their daily performances, particular cultural myths, myths that establish a dominant 'truth' as being 'natural to reality'. This second myth of a natural, objective reality is operating in all three case studies. The informants relayed symbols of bodily, physical, and mental differences as naturally occurring. Valorization, or the process by which these truths attain cultural value, is part of the process of simulation. It seems that the folk terms from the study help to show how signs mask reality and then, according to Baudrillard (1994), 'go on to mask the absence of reality'. For example, the idea that there is no difference, in a professional sense, between the two sexes would be well on its way to becoming a myth, if it were not for the way nursing culture is influenced by patriarchy and Maleness. This raises the important point that, in nursing culture, the *use value* of skills, as mentioned in the previous section, can be seen to be more about *sign value*. For simulation to occur, cultural meaning is organised around *consumption*, as opposed to the typical assumption of *production*. Thus, the representation of the symbolic body is for the viewer of the symbol. If the performance was 'good', then status identity is awarded. It is not *vice versa*, as the second myth may imply. For example, maleness incites a cultural meaning that promotes the 'strength' of men, the 'emotional detachment', 'aggression' and 'logic' that all men are [supposedly naturally] blessed with. These 'gender regime' type traits (Connell, 1987) can be seen as maleness providing symbols of commodity. The (re)production of performance needs consumption. If we assume that this were the truth and not a comical satire, then the symbolic body as a type of status would be widely accepted and obvious. Women would be the absent opposition, as argued by Kristeva (1982), and no longer needed for their [naturally occurring] caring and nurturing nature. Reputations have been won and lost on this limit boundary; boundaries, described by Connell, as cathexis and the social control and regulation of individuals and groups.

Despite the ludicrous appearance of this proposition, it has cultural meaning in psychiatric nursing culture. Data, taken from transcripts and observation journals, show how male nurses perceive themselves and are perceived as being more 'logical', 'emotionally redundant', 'dynamic', 'organised', 'pro-active', 'leaders of men', 'able to get things done', and' a figure head', to name just a few. Regardless of whether these folk terms were intended to be derogatory, it is still the case that male nurses are viewed differently due to these [naturally] occurring biological attributes. This defining of maleness, in the biological sense, is the symbolic body status reserved for the body with a penis. It is a status unobtainable by anyone without one and, therefore, women represent a limit of the male symbolic order. Femininity is a justification used by male nurses to defy this symbolic order and maintain 'their right to choose', to be 'autonomous', and be thought of as 'individual subjects', with personal trait characteristics that differ between men. The male body and persona is symbolic: it produces representations of what it is to be a male nurse. It provides a different identity and, therefore, a different status for male nurses. Male nurses have an identity that is not truly autonomous because, as subjects rather than individuals, all male nurses are trapped in the representations they are expected to perform. These representations are those that have a *simulated valid cultural meaning*.

Remembering Buchbinder (1998), 'the boundary willed by the male body has two purposes. First, it prevents the incursion of the outside world and second, 'it seals in' those menacing emotions from finding expression in, and blending with, the outside world. In opposition, the female body is a gateway. It is penetrable, weak and subject to desire'. Although this novel suggestion at first appears to be too psychoanalytic, it does carry some relevant notions that relate to the discovery of the status ethnographic, cultural themes. It is partly on the definition of the male body (as complete, closed and whole) that the subjectivity bestowed on men by patriarchy rests. The symbolic body is objectifiable; it can be 'gazed upon', as the male nurse is watched, and is also a spectator. In this sense, the body, as a status object, defies the possibility of individual identity for men and, thus, supports the earlier proposition that they are trapped in their representations.

'...we all nurse differently...If we were all the same, then it would be a really boring world wouldn't it' [Laughs].

(Stephen; Case 2 Interviews)

This is a common view shared by many of the men interviewed. It is perceived to be a truth, a natural truth that exists independently of man's meddling. The male nurses have a shared identity related to the sameness of their bodies, an identity categorised through a naturalising process. In terms of Buchbinder's claims above, the implicit nature of a closed body, which is strong and defensive, implies that men are, in a sense, a special gender, symbolised by specific representations and performances that justify and qualify their existence, within the realms of male identity. However, as proposed by all of the informants (including Stephen, above), nursing discourse proposes that men are gender-less in terms of their nursing identity because nursing, typically, promotes a gender-less cultural knowledge or, at least, does not promote cultures that expand gender representation, as referred to by John:

> 'I think nurses are nurses. There isn't a conspiracy to be any better, but to improve things generally...you know, there are good male nurses and there are good female nurses'

> (Case 3; Interviews)

This leads one to think that the impact of maleness is, perhaps, not so much of an impact because, if it were, it would be very recognisable.

There are at least two possible ways of analysing this. First, that there are a number of competing discourses, at least two of which we know, maleness and nursing. These can be seen to be constantly competing to maintain a status quo. Alternatively, it can be viewed that maleness is a splinter of the most dominant discourse (nursing) due to its inseparable nature from our biology, but it works by hiding itself within the 'technologies of the self and 'sites of representation' (Foucault, 1980) that nursing cultures provide. This book argues that the latter is the case, but does not deny that there are many competing discourses of which nursing is one.

Maleness is able to promote the gender-less representation in nursing culture because it is often thought to be special, as the universal and natural, a biological trait difference that just has to be accepted The only *difference* between the sexes in nursing is seen to be that of a biological nature. No other difference is relevant for discussion less an ugly 'truth' is discovered that cannot be smothered. The identity of the body is easily manipulated into both minoritising and universal views, i.e., how to be and how not to be. This dot-to-dot, or 'nursing by numbers', ethos enables male nurses to assume that the humanistic and existential belief in individual essence is true to their everyday reality. They chose to be who they are and maintain that certain identities are unthinkable and, therefore, have no place in the system On the other hand, as argued here, the thought that the cultural knowledge of nursing only allows a limited type of identity is often rejected. As speculated by Connell (1987) and, to an extent, Buckbinder (1998), these identities include those that can be penetrated. The feminine and the homosexual 'constitute the abject in patriarchy'. When exploring the body as status, we find a system of relationships that is not merely of difference, but rather of self-definition through difference, and this reminds us that the body as a status object defies the possibility of individual identity because subjects are trapped in the representation of signs.

What are the physical ways in which things are different for women?

> 'On the whole there's not a lot in it. Lifting, bending all that stuff has to be done regardless doesn't it? As a rule, we all do the same. There's no problem with that. It could be insulting to do all of the lifting, you know. We all take care to make sure our backs are OK.'

(Pat; Case 3 Interviews)

The following few paragraphs explore the way that most of the nurse informants assume masculinity exists in isolation from femininity. Women in the traditional sex type model can be seen as being constructed as 'minus male'; an absurd identity related to the symbolism and identity of the male body. This insight from post-feminist theory requires a broadening of the typically narrow inspection of gender issues. Nursing openly promotes certain norms of behaviour, while covering up innately human issues by excluding them. Yet, the symbolic male body in nursing survives as a concept. In fact, just being a nurse denies males a certain status. The low number of men in general nursing (approximately 10–12%; Royal College of Nursing, 1985) suggests that nursing is still considered a female occupation, one that requires the sensitive, caring, and nurturing skills, so often stereotyped as being representative of female nurses. According to Pontin (1988), the recruitment and study of men has been 'ignored for far too long', which reminds the reader of the continuing ambivalence to the study of gender issues in the nursing profession. The profession seems to keep such issues firmly tucked away under the hemline.

This brings to the forefront an assumption that all male nurses have to defend and rationalise in many experimental ways related to the symbolism and reputation of their body. The assumption is that being a male nurse requires a higher level of feminine characteristics than the average male in a non-nursing profession. This has consequences for identity in terms of status. The probability that male nurses over compensate male characteristics serves to emphasise the traditional linear, bi-polar model (of masculinity/femininity) favoured within nursing culture. This type of cultural knowledge acknowledges the status symbolism of the male body as occupying one end of a continuum and female traits another, and never the twain should meet.

However, from the start of the interviews, it became apparent that the male nursing world does not function as this linear model of difference would suggest. The issues related to maleness form a model resembling more of a web shape. In defence of their perceived reality (a linear model of difference), the men inadvertently provided alternative meanings of what it is like to be a male nurse; i.e., the resistance they have as individual social actors and the institutional assumptions of the nursing profession to view genders as anything but linear. The pressure male nurses describe in order to present themselves as in control is of particular relevance to the use of the male body as status in the company of other male colleagues. This is described by Bob (*Case 3 Interviews*):

> *'I'll tell you two things that I do that I try not or should learn not to do, but I still do it. One is to walk with the...err...prison officers roll. I don't know that I do it or how I got into the habit of*

doing it. It's not something I do, or did until somebody pointed it out to me...err...but it's a way of passing time and it's quite relaxing so you sort of rock back on the hips, rolling gait, a bit like an elderly sailor. I find I do that on the unit sometimes and I also quite consciously broaden my shoulders.'

Bob is not alone in his attempt to consciously make himself appear larger and more masculine, as described by James (*Case 3 Interviews*):

Do you think that having a male around is important?

Oh yes, It's a must isn't it. At the end of the day it's about safety and I see myself as providing that. Without the male staff I think that things would be chaos, because I wouldn't expect a female nurse to have to do what we have to do you know. When a big guy is angry and throwing chairs about it's important to get in there and put an end to it.

Masculinity does not exist in isolation from femininity—it will always be an expression of the current image men have of themselves in relation to women. At any given moment, gender identities will reflect the material interests of those who have power, and those who do not. Thus, relationships between men and women can be seen as politically constructed. This binary opposition is a central theme that runs throughout this book. It will appear again. It is argued that it is a sensible quest if only to illuminate the fact that studying differences between gender traits does not address the underlying issues related to social relations between men and women. Thus, the extracts just given express a concern by male nurses to try and keep the identity and male status afforded to them by society at large. The way to do this is by reinforcing the notion that there are differences and characteristics, which only men can do—usually because of physical attributes—that requires their presence within the wards.

Chapter 4
The symbols of maleness are active

'... men are expected to be tough and task orientated in our society, they should be harder, more competitive'.

Carol Watson (1997, p147)

'... We're all the same, male nurses just hang around the edges of any incident and let the females try and talk them down. It's only if things start to get out of hand we act.'

James (Male Nurse)

Dominance and prestige

Connell (1987) states that femininities are formed in the context of the 'global subordination of women to men'. The most common form is 'emphasised femininity'. This form of femininity is orientated to accommodating the interests and desires of men. This is a typical assumption made today as a result of the feminist theory of the last thirty years. It is an assumption based upon the issue of power, difference and, once again, the notion of the individual having agency. Although recognising that this type of argument is mainstream, it can also be useful to view the relationship between masculinity and femininity as a binary opposition. A structure that relies on contrast (difference).

The starting point for understanding maleness lies, not necessarily in the contrast with femininity, but in the asymmetric dominance and prestige that accrues to male nurses (via signs) in their nursing cultures. The idea of dominance and prestige has cultural meaning; it is thought of as being unsightly, yet assumed to be the way of the world. Most informants acknowledge its existence (the young newly qualified nurse who will trample over his colleagues to get promotion; the demanding charge nurse who insists that care plans are evaluated daily; in days gone by, the stout, no nonsense matron) yet, there is an emphasis that it is the responsibility of each individual to ensure that they do not enact this behaviour, as highlighted by Bill (*Case 3 Interviews*):

> '...*I'm not a pushy person, but I do want to get to the top. ... I don't think this is a bad thing. I think that in today's climate there is a pressure for everyone to do well...*'

The idea that Bill intimates is one recognised by most of the informants. Other male nurses spoke about 'feeling small', 'not knowing what they were doing', and 'being shouted at' by more senior staff, including doctors. These all have a bearing on the discussion of status, particularly that of dominance. It seems that there was a golden period of dominance in nursing, thought of by some as being part 'of the good old days' when matron ran 'a tight ship', as mentioned by Gary (*Case 3 Interviews*):

> '...*I can still remember the days when matron ran a tight ship. In those days you did as you were told...You know, you got to work on time.*'

The dominant ideology is not always the same. The 'good old days of matron' diminished and, with her departure, the advent of traditional nursing officers attempted to perpetuate the notion of order and rigidity. The meaning of dominance for male nurses has a more sinister side even though ideologies may arise, flourish and decay. Gary notes:

> '...*When I was younger it used to bother me that I was only a student, or just a staff nurse... you know, always being pushed around and told what to do. I'm very careful now to make sure that I'm not the same...*'

> '...*I think in those days that, as a man, it was sometimes very difficult to accept that you have to take orders from a woman.*'

> '...*I don't know, I think that other men probably felt the same as me. Status is something that you have to earn isn't it. Matron earned her status by fear.*'

Likewise, younger and less experienced male nurses knew about dominance and prestige as Liam (*Case 3 Interviews*) explained:

'...The ward manager tells us all what to do. Some of us joke about the way she should have been a man...Years ago it was like this all the time.'

The meaning of status, as represented by male nurses, is an encoded system of prescriptions and proscriptions about how to (re)produce maleness. It is deemed OK to accept orders from a respected older male nurse without any difficulty. But, in order to maintain a complete sense of 'self' (dignity) and an intact identity when being told what to do by a younger, less experienced, male staff nurse or female staff nurse, it is necessary to reluctantly follow orders and stress the differences. Yet, although the notion of men dominating women was a commonly included term of the study, it was always denied; a psychoanalytical understanding of the Oedipal [the Oedipal Myth], and Lacan (1968) would emphasise cultural forces harbouring hidden desires and wishes, for example, that male nurses dominate other male nurses and that the system is reflective of the subconscious. The myth being that male nurses assume, through individual diligence, they will be 'better', 'worth more', 'earn more by doing agency', and, by 'playing by the rules' get to 'the top', thus ensuring their status and dreaming their [individual] destiny. They do this by being active (re)producers of status behaviours; they masquerade as something that has cultural knowledge, thus providing status.

Active (re)producers

The notion of individuality as an agency is a powerful nursing discourse that encompasses maleness, as having an impact on the nature of status and identity in nursing cultural knowledge. But therein lies the third myth: male nurses are active (re)producers rather than passive producers of gender behaviours. As students, they learn to nurse in a male way; they develop and hone in on certain signs and abilities to perform the expected representations of maleness. This continues throughout their careers, as they attempt to limited or expand the (re)production of their gender behaviours to suit their particular masquerades at any given time. For example, the way

Anthony (*Case 3 Interviews*) describes the meaning of rituals, and the way these relate to moving on 'up through the ranks', reminds us of the institution of the army or other organisations:

> '...*I've been nursing for six years and I'm a staff nurse. That's considered all right, but in ten years time I'd look as though I was crap or something if I was still in the same post.*'

> '...*It's important that you keep trying to improve your skills and reputation so that you can move up through the ranks.*'

To be an active (re)producer, is to perform behaviours that have cultural knowledge, as representations of male traits. In order to do this, one has to be aware of the cultural knowledge and, therefore, subjected to it. Without cultural knowledge, there is no meaning. The constant (re)production, rather than being just the mere production of certain individual traits, is an idea that emphasises the way male nurses are subjectified into and by the maleness discourse: *representation is everywhere, it enables us to 'recognise particular versions of ourselves'* (Buchbinder, 1998). It provides us with a template from which male nurses can (re)produce a particular type of nursing; a male nursing that is aggressively denied as existing, but, nonetheless, entertains a certain gendered space. The notion of (re)production cheapens the original in the same way that a work of art is cheapened. It symbolises 'the same'; an identical array of skills, approaches and attitudes. If we consider the psychiatric nursing cultures of the large hospitals in the UK, we can see that divergence and difference is not abundant. This emphasises the way that male nurses continue to (re)produce rather than produce identity, and the view of Baudrillard (1994) that consumption is not just an economic and material activity, but also a symbolic (meaningful) and status differentiating activity. This rebukes the sex type gender theorists, such as Moir and Moir (1999), Lemkau (1984) and Bem (1974), as concentrating excessively on production at the expense of consumption. Thus, identity as active (re)production and consumption is coded with secondary level connotation meaning, smothered with hidden messages of myth.

Some may argue that advancing nursing practice and pushing the boundaries of clinical care is an organisational-/evidence-based process that is not achievable, the responsibility of the individual, or, alternatively, that change takes time and cannot be immediate. In response to these suggestions, the researcher argues that the expectations made of male nurses change as the larger ideological structures permit. Even though history is dotted with great figures who have, seemingly, single-handedly changed the history of world, with mature understanding, we recognise that this linear model is seldom the case, regardless of the significance 'of work' in the construction of gender identity, as argued by Tolson (1977). Change and advancement occurs when the performance of representations in the expectations of cultural knowledge allow for change.

By insisting that masculinity and its binary opposite, femininity, are naturally occurring entities, a current dominant social organisation of people is perpetuated and protected, and a particular construction of the world preserved: a construction that gives the body a status of determining how social actors should behave. Such an obvious statement has been easily misunderstood to mean that females cannot be fathers, or be independent; they are fickle, emotional and need protecting (from other men by men). Of course, the safety of such a construction can be realised when we consider that *(i) we are also given identity,* and *(ii) we are able to find our place in the social structure.* The body gives us an identity, a status, and an excuse/reason why we should want/need to be socially dominant, particularly if you have a penis. In this sense, male nurses are all biological and ideological subjects, and the culture of nursing is no exception to this. The cultural meaning of maleness and status in nursing is related to gender theory only in so far as it has an emic quality to the informants: namely, that it is the *sex written on the body.* This makes the body legible to the culture in particular ways, and subject to the requirements of the dominant gender myths. The process of identity begins with the body as a subject.

In the following chapter, this theory is extended to show how the focal data of the study provides reasonable evidence to suggest that the notion of (re)production, as discussed, has a direct relationship to 'the performance of self'. And how individuals are *subjectified* by the discourse of maleness, as it impacts on the cultural knowledge to which they contribute. Once again, the majority of informants from the three case studies emphasised the notion of the autonomous and free thinking individual with personality traits, as being at 'the centre'. The researcher will argue that there is enough focal data to propose that the individual is absent and 'decentred'.

Chapter 5
Vulnerability is a result of maleness

'Feminists like Dworkin and Mackinnon place an absolute premium on the autonomy of the self, which for them resides above all in the 'privacy of the body'.'

Tom Morton (1997, p161)

'Sometimes we're put in vulnerable situations'.

Simmy (Male Nurse)

Introducing the performance of symbols

Male nurses perform specific representations of maleness that 'create tension in the subjective positions' in which they find themselves (Buchbinder, 1998 ; Tolson, 1977). For most of the male informants, this can be likened to the included term 'vulnerability', a cover term that has within it a number of themes not usually associated with masculinity (at least not in public). Yet, in private, there is—even if at only a pseudo level—a recognition that male nurses are subject to conditions that require a particular way, i.e., a male way, of dealing with the worry of having no choice, but to perform maleness. For most, this amounts to 'it not feeling right', or 'needing to follow one's heart', as opposed to a recognition that they are subject to discursive phenomena. The following three sections provide evidence to suggest that:

1. Repeated performance maintains a constant unchanging sign of identity for consumption;

2. Subjectivization can occur without the subjects' knowledge or consent;

3. The performance of male nurses is about a subjectivized identity;

4. This performance is about adhering to the rituals, rules and scripts of Maleness. This being trapped in representation is the penalty of subjectivization;

5. In psychiatry this can be seen in the use of intimacy as a professional performance; and

6. Vulnerability is linked to an inability to be an active performer at a conscious level.

For a male to be burdened with the shame of 'not being able to manage his ward', there is a strong symbolism and performance anxiety. It is deemed reasonable or even 'natural' (and, therefore, expected) for female nurses to react differently to stress; to get 'hysterical' and 'upset', as discussed in myth no 3 in the previous section. But such an outburst by male nurses is seen to undermine the standard performance required of maleness. To perform maleness legitimately, you have to be able to deal with everything and anything that, as one informant said, 'is thrown at you', but, just as important, you have to 'do it like a man'. You have to perform maleness that is worthy of the intended representation. This type of gender representation (as understood by the researcher when observing the informants) appeared to be linked: first, to fear and anxiety; second, to keeping up appearances; and third, to competition. This allegiance to masculinity seemed to be intrinsically combined to the character of performance. This section has two aims related to the process of subjectivization of male nurses. First, to clarify what is meant by vulnerability, as a cultural meaning for the male informants, and second, to develop the thesis related to the subjectivization of male nurses by maleness. In particular, the way maleness determines the 'performance of the self', as opposed to individuals having an autonomous self.

Cultural meaning is for the weak

Men are active; they are doers; they control their own world; indeed, they control the natural world; they don't cry; and they certainly don't talk about it if they do. They play with an emotional poker face everyday; and they never get emotionally close enough to be hurt.

If all of this were really true, then one imagines that male nurses have some very easy rules to follow. It would also be plausible to suspect that, in private, male nurses acted a different Goffmanian (1959) type performance, i.e., a different presentation of their daily self. Male nurses deny that the structure promoting the (re)production of these stereotypes impacts on them to such an extent that they are relieved of their individual autonomy, and are subjectivized. Furthermore, their sense of ontology is not one of existential anxiety-ridden essences and humanist inner cores, but one of repeated performances shaped by the maleness discourse, which presents the illusion that they, as individuals, can maintain the constant unchanging *identity* previously discussed. There is a cultural myth (myth number 4) that male nurses (as caring professionals) are more in touch with their 'feminine side' and probably more able than other occupational groups to have [(re)produce value signs for consumption] 'emotional' traits. The ethnographic theme highlights the meaning that this 'being emotional' is a carefully orchestrated ideology with many connotations. The decentred male nurse uses performance, or to be more exact, consistent performances, not only to provide him with a *status identity*, but also to maintain and naturalise the myth of the feminine *performance*.

By doing field work in a psychiatric unit, it can be observed that male nurses view themselves as 'good listeners', as 'instinctively knowing when a patient needs interaction'; many of the male nurses reported that they were *'people* people' that is, they came into nursing to help people. Nevertheless, it can be observed that these same nurses also consider themselves 'in control', 'calm' and 'able to maintain boundaries'. Such boundaries signify what is just too emotional, and defend against 'taking work too seriously', 'getting wound up', and in need of a structured and logical male distance. Any male nurse who is perceived to be 'over involved' is vulnerable. Any male nurse who does not adhere to the unit boundaries is taking a risk. Any male nurse who crosses the line of professionalism is in the same dangerous category as the rapist, sexual pervert, or a 'woolly woofter'. Hence, the freedom of choice, the liberty of agency that has been introduced in the preceding few sections can be seen to be at the mercy of institutional rituals, politics, and rules for the utilitarian good of all. These defences and taboos are there to protect; they are structures added on to the culture and stand as ideological guardians against the horrors of practice committed in days gone by.

This is all part of a larger discourse that warns against the sexual nature of man, and his inability to resist temptation when forming close trust relationships. Arguably, it is an albatross hanging around all psychiatric nursing cultures. Male nurses adhere to specific rituals and rules as prescribed by cultural knowledge, but they do so because they are vulnerable if they do not. They are vulnerable because, at a practical level, cultural knowledge defends the established norms and will not tolerate any male nurse who dares to publicly challenge traditional representations. As noted by Mahony (1999) in a nursing article entitled: *'Men behaving badly'*, 'there's no disguising the fact that many more males than females go before UKCC conduct hearings'. The statistics show that male nurses make up just 9% of the nursing register, but have been involved in 48% of conduct hearings (Mahony, 1999). The cultural norms that enforce an expected type of male nursing are seen to be there for the protection of the public. Male nurses live with the legacy of temptation, sexual urges, and the need to be policed and police themselves.

Allegiance to masculinity

The principle of conformity is to yield to group pressures. In exchange theory, this is termed as social pressure. Pressure is viewed as impacting on 'the individual'. This dominant perspective about the nature of power is the myth that has cultural knowledge, and is known by all nurses within psychiatric nursing cultures. This is knowledge and power to inhibit and prevent action of individuals to break the group consensus. It is also emphasised by informants that variety is welcomed in the expressions, such as 'live and let live' and 'each to his own'. It is assumed that a dynamic and living culture (as a type of reflection of democratic liberalism) is able to absorb such deviance as a function that creates healthy change within a culture's internal systems. However, if such an idyllic culture exists, it is not within psychiatric nursing. The very existence of the ethnographic domain: 'Vulnerability is a result of maleness', indicates that all is not as it is romantically presented by the informants.

The opposite of this conformity model could be the case: there is no knowledge of such conformity without cultural meaning. The inconsistency presented by the informants in statements, such as, 'each to his own' on the one hand, and getting too 'emotionally close' on the other, indicates that larger ideological structures are at work, structures that have the power to regulate social conduct and disguise it as natural. Like some great conspiracy, the meaning of vulnerability for the male informants seems to be based upon a pre-decided script, which each of them stuck to as though being interrogated. So what does this mean? It seems to suggest that it is very difficult for male nurses to admit to being vulnerable, to being just a little bit human, as opposed to being the machine - like nurses churned out by too many schools of nursing. Male nurses have cultural knowledge of their units, of their role, and the expected representations, because their subjectivity, their position in the discourse constitutes the 'knowledge' that male nurses represent non-vulnerability.

Male nurses have allegiance to masculinity, because their subject position is embedded within it. The maleness discourse subjectivizes them from day one in the school of nursing. The myths (openly shared cultural beliefs) of masculinity and nursing reside in the maleness discourse. Bodily attributes and capacities, such as emotional detachment, behaviour, and withdrawal are acquired through the 'brute outcome' of imitation and doing (consider myth 3: subjects are active (re)producers). Both the interview and observation data suggest that 'learning the ropes', 'watching others', and 'gaining experience' have cultural meaning for all the nurse informants. They perceive that pre-existing practice is the natural and best way to do nursing and male nurses work in certain ways that are comparable to their female colleagues. In other words, the notions of vulnerability work upon male nurses, subjectifying them, 'without necessarily winning them over in the head' (Nixon, 1997).

If we are suggesting that male nurses are vulnerable, as a result of their subject positioning, are they really vulnerable at all? Surely, the fact that they are representing the dominant ideologies of masculinity in nursing obscures the possibility that they are in some way vulnerable? The answer lies in the fact that all male nurses are subjectivized to represent maleness because they are constituted by maleness. They are vulnerable to (re)producing the wrong maleness in terms of the myths of masculinity and nursing. One hug too many, one tear, one over zealous restraint (let alone one accusation of sexual misconduct) makes them vulnerable to not performing maleness correctly. They become answerable to the charge of mis-representing maleness, which will disassociate itself by the power/knowledge it holds within the culture; that is, it will blame the individual subject and protect the discourse. The transcript below (*Simmy Case 3*) hides within it these real everyday vulnerabilities:

> *'Ummm...well when you work in an environment which is mostly female like this, where the vast majority of patients are female, ummm...I feel like a second rate nurse. I get fed up with not being able to be part of the routine, you know like escorts and I'm always the one who does the drugs...I'm conscious of the boundaries between the older male nurse and the female patients. I'm very conscious that I have to be very sure of the situation. Sometimes we're put in vulnerable situations because young girls fall in love...you know. That's why I have to be very conscious of the boundaries and also the issue of checking through the property and that, plus going off the ward with female patients. These restrict me.'*

What Simmy is explaining is his ideological view of reality. Young female patients fall in love with him, older male nurses get easy job, and his world is surrounded by females. He, like all the male informants, acknowledged that his 'performance of self' is defined by appropriate boundaries of interaction. Perhaps the argument that it is the subject-position that provides the conditions for individuals to act, or have 'knowledge' in relation to particular social practices, is one worthy of consideration. In this case, knowledge enough to know that 'falling in love with a patient', 'crying with a patient', or 'seeking too much supervision' can be seen as a weakness, because male nurses in psychiatry 'need to be self-contained' and 'dependable'. Remembering the included terms related to the comment: 'we work as a team' and 'if you can't rely on your colleagues, who can you rely on?' reminds us that male nurses are ideologically programmed to be warm, honest, and genuine in the humanist sense, but they remain unaware that they occupy a particular subject-position.

The representation of biological sex role traits of male nurses mark the formation of new subject-positions for men. They are at the very edge of **not** what it is to be an individual, a human with emotions and weakness, but at the boundary of cultural myths related to masculinity and nursing. The advent of the 'new man' is symbolised by the male nurse, as he juggles with the seemingly endless possibilities that amount to only one: his [repeated] *performance* of self as determined by his discursive subject-position. 'Vulnerability is a result of maleness' is a domain that allows for an examination of the emergence of more contemporary forms of individuality, through the growth of new bodies of knowledge and networks of power. This domain highlights male nurses' allegiance to the myths of masculinity, due to their inescapable relationship with their subject positioning by the maleness discourse. Paradoxically, this is most commonly associated with male nurse's abilities to use 'the [autonomous] self' in the representation of 'intimacy', 'a caring attitude', or as an 'expression of their feminine side'. This will now be discussed.

Male intimacy

As with Simmy in his earlier extract, the meaning of vulnerability, as an all exclusive cover term, compromises two typical responses. First, there are those, like Simmy's, which indicated anxieties surrounding direct patient care, in case it exposes the carer to inclusion in the sex/pervert categories.

Second, the responses associated with being sued for bad practice. These responses all remain outside the emotional. The informants never offered responses that indicated a sense of fear, loneliness, upset, or panic; instead, they offered anger, frustration, and problem-solving. Attributes, such as anger and problem solving, are usually associated with masculine biological traits, as opposed to the feminine characteristics. Thus, the cultural meaning of vulnerability seemed to replicate the ideological expectations. What this indicates is the possibility that male nurses find themselves in subject-positions that attempt to protect certain ideologies and these, in turn, legitimise male action: correctly represented action born from an awareness of cultural knowledge.

The work of Hite (1987; 1994), using qualitative surveys and interviews, is well-known for being at the forefront of issues of relationships and intimacy between the sexes. The focal data of this study supports her themes and patterns regarding the nature of male intimacy. This is because the language and myths that shape peoples lives belong to closed systems of discourse. The maleness discourse promotes the dominant ideologies prevalent in wider society. We have the means to argue that, over the past twenty years, there has been an emergence of new knowledge about the subjectivity of the male experience. It is no longer considered a 'no go area', or one that is assumed to be commonsense. Male intimacy is big business. Adverts, chat shows, Internet problem pages and men only chat rooms all signify the dawn of a new era, one not only acknowledging the fact that males have worries, but also that some men want to share their experiences. This reiterates the call by Tolson (1977) that males need a supportive space in which to learn to share experiences. The nursing discourse promotes a sense of professionalism, individuality, and order before all other ideologies. As such, the typical notions of male intimacy are exposed, as being about professional performance, as opposed to a masculine one. The following extract is from Bob (*Case 3 Interviews*) :

> '*I used to help a young lady get dressed every morning, through the entire procedure of putting everything on, and this was a really good way to earn a living. And I wasn't fully aware, or fully*

prepared for it. And...urm...it certainly was very interesting being the male worker in this all female environment.'

'...You didn't go into the female dormitory...umh...unless there was nobody in there, especially in a state of undress. You could go in if people were just resting and call a patient out. And you'd have to go in sometimes because the linen cupboard was placed in there...'

This account shows how the meaning of vulnerability is linked to an inability to be an active performer, or to be an active subject. Vulnerability for male and female nurses does not have different meanings, just different intensities (Gary, *Case 3 Interviews*):

'I not really sure...erm...I think there may be certain aspects or facets to my role which probably equate to examination of female patients, the body domain of nursing I think would distinguish my role from that of my female colleagues. This has never really proved to be a problem and I often find that most patients really don't mind whether they get a male or female nurse to look after them and I think they're quite happy and I've certainly never had any problems.'

What is the nature of intimacy for male nurses? It seems to have something to do with 'keeping a safe distance', yet not admitting this could ever be the case, because this would negate the male role, perhaps, as being secondary to female nurses. Such an assumption is based upon the premise that intimacy is an important nursing tool in the welfare of their patients. To be able to be intimate, yet professional, seems to be the knife edge that male nurses perch on daily during their many interactions with patients. This can be related to the experience just given in Bob's extract. Man to man interaction seems to be about upholding the value of masculinity. To be intimate does not allow this. In fact, masculinity does not allow this. Being a joker and 'having a laugh' are typical strategies employed by male nurses, sometimes without even realising it, to avoid intimate interactions with their patients.

In terms of what intimacy means for the male informants, it seems that the words get stuck in the throat of each one. It is very difficult for a male nurse to express intimacy, as a therapeutic tool, without the fear of being branded a sexual pervert. This is the professional boundary cultural 'meaning' that has been discussed previously. Hence, the difference between male and female nurses. But such an assertion is denied by the male informants, who dismissed intimacy as a reliable or valid therapeutic procedure to help their patients regain health (myth 1 and 2). This idea of sexuality shares a distinct relationship with the 'meaning' of intimacy for male nurses. A collection of extracts helps to demonstrate this assertion:

Simmy (Case 3 Interviews):

> '*Umm…I can always remember when I was a student nurse on a medical ward and umm…there was this young female patient, I think she was only about twenty-two and urm…I was asked to give her a suppository, I think, but, nowadays, I wouldn't do that.*

Pat (Case 3 Interviews):

> '*Well errr…I wouldn't let male students get the female patients up in the morning and that, and I think that all nurses would agree with that, even the females. It's an ethical thing isn't it…*

Bill (Case 3 Interviews):

> '*Yeah, you know…looking after female patients and that, it's obvious that male nurses need to care for females in the same way that female nurses have to look after male patients, but there's a difference in outlook isn't there…Most of the general public couldn't imagine a female nurse doing anything sexual, [i.e. sexual contact with a patient] whereas a male nurse would be accused because he was a male…'*

Performing subject positions

To ensure that the following chapter makes sense (power and hierarchy, which focus on the issue of *individuality*), this section aims to draw together the discussion so far. Up to this point, there has been a concern with introducing the reader to the idea of maleness, as a term relating to the myths and discourse that impact upon male nurses (in terms of subjectivization) and nursing culture. Both myths and discourse are terms used to denote ideologies. These ideologies can be analysed in terms of the mythical 'truths' they uphold or disregard in any cultural knowledge. For example, this discussion has argued, so far, that all nurses are subjects in discourse and exposed to myths promoting universalism, essentialism, biological determinism, and free will.

The evidence to support the existence of these myths resides in the data collected during the study; evidence suggesting that nurses are 'subjectivized', and that being a subject of discourse has ontological implications on *identity* (status) and *performance* (vulnerability). It can be seen that the status theme introduces what the notion of identity is for the mental health nurses, and how this conflicts with the semiotic theory applied by the researcher. In these sections on vulnerability and performance, the concern has been to show how performance of maleness identity creates performance anxieties, as male nurses (re)produce representations. The following chapters will bring to an end the discussion of subjectivization by taking the discussion into the area often associated with humanism: *individuality*. Before that, it is necessary to make a number of crucial theoretical points so that no misunderstanding can occur.

Maleness discourse and myths requires nurses to identify a particular configuration of signs as signifying maleness, a recognition that, at the same time, interpellates males as ideologically obedient subjects, i.e., as masculine. However, as noted by Buchbinder (1998: p121), even though such signs may, at first, appear evident and beyond question, we should note that sign systems may prove dangerous in their signifying capability. The development of myths shows that the constellation of signs can be read as signifying other 'meanings' in addition to the preferred one. This can be extended to the observer, as an 'excess of signification' as symbols are consumed (Baudrillard, 1994). The key element is repetition of signs: in this case repeated signs of gender as performances, the most dominant of which are shown in *Figure 5.1*.

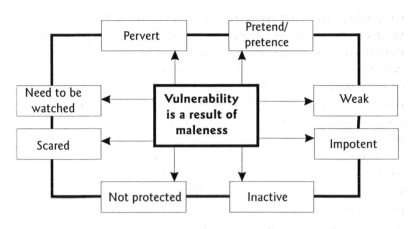

Figure 5.1: The most dominant signs of gender as performances

This has introduced the notion that there are no naturally occurring gender traits and, as such, argued against the sex type nursing theorists cited in *Chapter One* (Ratcliffe, 1996; Smith, 1993; James, 1992; Robinson, 1992; Hesselbart, 1977; Hoffman, 1970), and, in particular, the insistence of Pontin (1988) that male nurses take on board feminine traits, but can still be 'differentiated from female nurses'. Male nurses can, indeed, do the same (re)production of signs as female nurses; they can even represent female nurses to a limited extent, but, as subjects, they have a gender position representing masculinity in which male nurses 'do maleness' ['do gender']. The fieldwork data enabled the author to identify the included terms of: 'having the experience', 'knowing what to do in an emergency', 'having an aura', 'by working hard', 'having authority to get things done', and 'being level headed'. These included terms were snippets of 'doing' gender through an array of observable signs and sign systems. The signs themselves are neither natural nor perpetual in their performance and use value.

The existence of maleness is, thus, hidden and with it, the cultural knowledge that male nurses are subjectivized. As shown by Barthes' (1996), 'myths' maleness is dissolved as a named identity through a naturalising process (myth 2), a process that can be seen to become the property of the individual as opposed to the subject. It becomes possible to illuminate the relationship between subject positions and the performative nature of gender, as a weak attribute that must be reinforced constantly and, hence, made visible in nursing culture, in order for subjects to maintain their *'individual'* sense of *identity*. At the same time, both maleness and nursing discourse seek to make that gender performance invisible, so that it appears natural and, hence, beyond question.

The data enables a thorough examination of psychiatric nursing culture's minoritising and universalising views. Every semantic relationship, included term, and taxonomy helps to emphasise the unstable *identity, performance,* and notion of the *individuality* that male nurses aspire to. But how do individuals account for this type of subjectivization? In the main, they do not know it is happening. All the nurse informants emphasised the role of the individual, a role that is seen to be responsible for constituting agency. Such agency is assumed to have a relationship with the cultural theme of power and hierarchy. This is the next step in the book concerning the subjectivization of nurses. The following chapters examine the way male nurses (encoded by their subjectivization) aim to empower themselves as autonomous *individuals*, by climbing the hierarchical ladder and competing as individuals against other individuals. Individuality (in male nurses: manliness) is, thus, defined for them unknowingly by the discourse of maleness and the myths that protect and hide its controlling existence. The experience of the 'identified performing individual', as highlighted in the data, indicates that male nurses operate under the assumption that they must show other men how they can succeed where others fail, professionally, personally, and sexually. Given this simulated reality, i.e., the performance of symbols for consumption that are inauthentic, and the additional burden of having to show more of a 'feminine side', it is hardly surprising that male nurses 'vulnerability' is centred on attempts to conceal or suppress elements that might betray them in cultural knowledge.

Chapter 6
He who has the hierarchy,
has the power

'The office is a formidable bastion of nursing power.
It has a row of IKEA chairs waiting for the handover.
These are framed by an equal number of glass panes through
which to exert power.'

Field Journal (Study 1; Day 1)

Power and hierarchy are used to do maleness

A person walking into a psychiatric ward for the first time will find it hard to locate a hierarchy. Everybody will be dressed similarly, so there is a lack of the most obvious hierarchical symbol, the uniform. However, it is possible, given time, to begin to define the symbols of hierarchy. For even in the most seemingly egalitarian of places, hierarchy and power relationships exist. They reside, not in the individual nurses, but in the culture as a web of knowledge and relationships. Yet all the nurse informants perceive power and hierarchy as 'something personal', something to do with a nurse's 'personality', 'experience', 'nursing grade', and the ability of individuals to 'climb to the top'.

It is the aim of the next four sections to argue that the data collected during the study supports the developing thesis already introduced. Specifically, that the issue of power and hierarchy is more about cultural knowledge and the social relationships between nurses who are 'subjects', rather than about 'individual' keepers of power. It is the subject, not the individual who wears the uniform. Hence, the fifth myth that concerns how power and *individuality* are actively promoted as masquerades of 'identity and performance' in the person-centred, humanistic, derived myths of maleness and nursing discourse :

1. Individuals do not have essential, universal or determined power;

2. Individuals have experience and qualifications that, in the social context, elevate them up the hierarchy. This affords them authority and power;

3. This simulation of personal attributes resides in the subject and role, as constituted in cultural knowledge and not in the individual;

4. In this way, the subject is decentred, as opposed to the individual being centred;

5. There are different subject positions within the decentred space. To belong to a marginalised subject position will mean a loss of power; e.g., being feminine, being gay, being suspected of either, of not being 'management material', 'not knowing the right people'; and

6. These appear to be the different tribes of maleness.

For many mental health nurses, there is a spoken belief that psychiatric wards are not hierarchical; that such pompousness is actively discouraged and left for 'the real nurses' [general nurses]. However, despite denials, these claims are not plausible. Bold hierarchies based on the traditional model of two senior nurse managers, two junior nurse managers, a body of trained nurses and a core of non-trained nurses function to give the illusion that this framework has authority and power. Yet, despite the denial of such hierarchies being central to how a ward functions (and the insistence that the individual practitioner is central), nurses will readily 'pass the buck' to more senior nurses when decisions need to be made; after all, 'they get paid for it'.

The concepts of hierarchy and power are sociological topics that have been well-researched and documented, as noted in *Chapter One*. It was expected that, during the study, these issues would emerge in certain guises as cultural symbols. The domain: 'Hierarchy is used to do maleness' emerged early and overlaps with many of the included terms positioned in the other five domains of maleness. It is an important theme because power and hierarchy are, fundamentally, social issues.They are cultural and go someway to define many facets of psychiatric nursing culture, particularly, the nature of what it is to be a 'powerful' male nurse.

It is plausible to suggest that the issue of power and hierarchy for male nurses is not so 'cut n' dry', even though the major issue of, 'Who was in charge?', 'Who was a good leader?' etc, are often reflected as being important in nursing culture. A primary consideration of this book (after the notion of identity) is the notion of *individuality*, symbolised, at its sharpest, by power and hierarchy. This emic (views of the nurse informants) 'individuality' is in direct contrast to the notion of nurses being in subject positions, i.e., individuality for the informants has denotations of agency, freewill, and autonomy to exercise individual power in order to achieve seemingly individually induced outcomes. Although the data could support this traditional exchange theory notion, the use of a semiotic perspective raises strong possibilities that, because individuals are being subjectivized (their cultural knowledge is constituted by discourse and seduced by myths), when they use 'power', they are not simply acting as autonomous beings, but rather, reinforcing the powerful structures that fix them in cultural knowledge. In this case, the structure is the maleness discourse as it operates within psychiatric nursing culture.

The two dominant sub-themes that emerged from the data to support this idea were: (i) *'Roles'—which allowed the (re)production of power*, and (ii) *Tribes (difference due to gender as opposed to sex/the idea of fragmented masculinities taken from Mac an Ghaill (1985) and Connell (1987) and developed in nursing culture with relevance to maleness)*. There are two points that need to be argued in order to provide a strong case for this book. First, to show that, for the informants, power and hierarchy, as common sociological concepts, have a typical emic 'cultural meaning' that relies on common signs and symbolism for its exchange. This informant view needs to be explored using focal data from the study. Second, to argue that power and hierarchy in psychiatric nursing culture is a product of cultural knowledge. That the domain, 'power and hierarchy, is used to do maleness' demonstrates how male nurses use (do not own or have individual) power and hierarchies and, therefore, contribute to the production of meaning using signs. The result being that maleness is represented and represents typical assumptions and stereotypes (which emphasises difference) usually associated with the two concepts.

Exploring the emic meaning (power and hierarchy)

The study of the relationship between gender and power continues to be a fashionable one, and has always been complicated by the debate over how research should be conducted. In many popular books about male issues, authors described a masculinity characterised by aggression, competitiveness, emotional ineptitude, and coldness. These are the typical cultural symbols noted in the previous sections regarding *identity* and the *performance* of the self. Likewise, the work of Jeffery Weeks (1981; 1985) emphasises the impact of what he called the sexual tradition in setting the big terms for the shaping of contemporary sexualities. These 'big terms' have traditionally played upon binary oppositions (e.g., men are active, women are passive) and emphasised how men have always had the power resources in all stratifications of society. It is with these assumptions (that are indeed the myths of psychiatric nursing culture) that the researcher encountered the cultural meanings associated with male nurses and power/hierarchy. This section will begin with an exploration of these assumptions and then, using the ethnographic sub themes, put forward a thesis produced using data from this study that applied a semiotic analysis of these traditional beliefs.

It is usual to begin by attempting to produce a single all-embracing conceptualisation of power. This is extremely difficult because power is assumed to exist in all human phenomena. Therefore, we ask the question: Which definition of power is most useful? There are so many to choose from. When asked, mental health nurses spoke about 'leadership', 'being in charge', and 'having responsibility' (see *Figure 6.1*). Each had its carefully constructed predictors, matrixes, and checklists to help nurses understand the type of manager they are, the type of personality they have, the likelihood of gaining promotion. In a world where all nurses are expected to (acquire a knowledge of such issues—and expect it of themselves), it is hardly surprising that cultural knowledge becomes entrenched in an obsession to find, secure, and establish a consensus; one that is based upon 'image' (the consistent visual sign) above all others.

Hierarchy	Status	Machoness
authority	leadership	masculine
'recognition'	experience	hard
'getting things done'	authority	non emotional
'having the qualifications'	'earned respect from similar grades'	opposite to feminine
'right place at the right time'	'know what you are doing'	bully
'more money'	'remaining calm'	strong body
'to get your own way'	'give advice'	expected
'work your way to the top'	'a sense of dignity'	defensive
'taking the flak'	'self-respect'	logical
'responsibility'	'respect from others'	loud
'give leadership and direction'	'listening'	dominant
'getting on with the work'	'being considerate'	boisterous
'institutional commitment'	'consistent interactions'	loyal
'brown nosing'	'a sense of achievement'	'fitting in'
'blagging'	'a sense of role'	'not being taken seriously'
'doing your share'	'status is a personal thing'	'by being a lad'
'an easy life'	'personality type'	'acting the fool'
'respect'	'confidence'	'loudly'
'figure head'	'not panicking'	'male chauvinists'
'an aura'	'putting on a front'	'telling dirty jokes'
'protect'	'can be relied on'	'by pretending to be something you're not'
'a good team player'	'being in pro-active alliances'	'a false front'
'duty to climb the ranks'	'doing the rough jobs'	'being like a man'
'sorting things out'	'keeping stumm'	'bouncing around—throwing your weight around'
'top of the tree'		'showing a lack of emotion'
		'not thinking'
		'having a laugh'
		'being one of the boys'
		'doing nothing'
		'being the opposite of what women do'
		'knowing what you're meant to be'
		'openly showing aggression'

Figure 6.1: Analysis of the three primary cover terms of Case 1

As with the theme of identity, the nurses in the case studies believe in a model of power that is individually centred, something which is tangible and seemingly real in their everyday experiences. Certain nurses have more power because they are higher in the hierarchy, some nurses have less because they are non-trained, and so on. There is also the idea that power and status within the hierarchy is dependent on what goes on inside the nurse's head. Examples indicate the way some informants perceive the ward around them and how many alliances they have to make with other influential nurses in 'high places'. The dominant belief is one putting forward the argument that, in nursing, individuals have power and status dependent upon the hierarchy. Even though it is possible to have status as a non-trained nurse, or certain power (authority to request from others) as a staff nurse, it is easier to establish these concepts as an *individual* attribute, if you are a higher grade nurse. This is the simple answer to the question: Which definition of power is most significant for psychiatric culture? However, it is not the definition this book argues.

The definition that each nurse informants brought with them to the interviews and gave during the observations were the emic definitions listed in the domains and taxonomies (see *Figure 6.1*). These reflect the assumptions postulated in the previous paragraph. From these, the author developed a cultural theme: it is not the **individual** who has power, but the culture in which s/he is situated. Power is sexless and fixes itself to cultural meaning of how maleness should be performed. This premise is best broken down into the following three points that synthesise important contributions of post-structural theory.

- Nurses can only have knowledge of things if things have cultural meaning. It is discourse, not the things in themselves that produce knowledge. Knowledge is put to work through discursive practices to regulate the conduct of others. The discourse of patriarchy and masculinity in nursing—maleness—produces a certain kind of knowledge that goes to regulate the performance, (re)production, representation, and simulation of signs

- Power operates within the limits of maleness, the assumption being that 'psychiatry needs men'. However, male nurses are not more powerful as subjects/individuals (than others); they are representing maleness, which is more powerful in power's circulation
- Power is productive in the constitution of maleness through specific visual codes and forms of looking. It fixes the boundaries between the normal and the abnormal (binary oppositions of maleness—that which is non-male).

What do these points mean? The answer continues in tandem with the ideas already introduced. All nurses belong to a culture. They understand this culture because objects, people, and events have cultural meaning. Meaning is exchanged via signs. These meanings are knowledge; typically, knowledge (myths/ideologies) at a *denotation* level that informs nurses how their ward should operate, how it has always operated, what belongs where and why. The *connotation* level is more about how they should behave and what the penalties will be if their conduct is wrong. This study in the first phase has been about discovering the emic denotation 'meaning' (e.g. what are all of the ways/uses of/results of/attributes of power and hierarchy). In the second place, it was concerned about interpreting the meaning and connotations that circulate in psychiatric nursing cultural knowledge. All nursing rituals and procedures are perceived to be based on denoted 'sound knowledge', i.e., the best knowledge and practice. However, every sign by definition also has ideological connotations. For example, the best type of nursing care is delivered by doing such and such; every 'good' nurse wants to give the 'best care' so they do it this way. The researcher lost count of the many times he heard 'we do it this way here because…'. These ideologies are not the only knowledge, but the dominant one. It is often assumed that the way things are done is because it is 'the best way' based on the 'best knowledge' (the commonsense way, etc). Yet knowledge is determined by power operating within institutional apparatus, rather than knowledge necessarily being 'the best' and determined by individual practitioners who are fulfilling research-based practice endorsed by nursing discourse. Likewise, male nurses, not the individual male nurse represent maleness, which has a powerful impact.

'The legend of the individual—the denial of the subject'

Roles—(re)producing power

Without wishing to stray from the central aim of discussing the issues of power and hierarchy, it is important to acknowledge the vast array of theories pertaining to what philosophers throughout the centuries (and more recently sociologists) consider to be 'the *individual*'. The idea that, as individuals, we have an inner self has, since the Renaissance, been taken for granted in argument. The premise for this book, however, is that individuality, as a concept, is not essential or constitutes agency, but rather a determined social construction that is interwoven into many social relationships and arrangements, based on dominant cultural knowledge. Therefore, the idea that groups of 'new age men' can spend an instinctive, naked weekend together in an attempt to return to nature and find the real 'inside' masculinity, as proposed by Bly (1992), is futile (even if it might be fun). All this will become more apparent, as we begin to see how the male nurses perceive their own individual power base and potential promotion in terms of the hierarchy they experience.

As indicated by the 'legend' musing introducing this section, it seems that having experience and a long-standing history enables male nurses to acknowledge the leaders of the pack. These leaders are often perceived to be very powerful because they have been true to 'themselves'. They are nurses who 'know their stuff' and 'are up for it'. When asked the question, 'What are the personal attributes used by male nurses to do hierarchy?', the answers fell into a single category of individual qualities. Informants gave answers, such as 'being a good leader', 'to have responsibility', 'seen to be in charge', 'the onus is on you', and many other responses typifying the assumption that the individual is central, contained, and separate to the wider organisational self; and that there is an inner core or essence (myth 1) 'the self' on which experience, authority, and skill can be layered as the years go by. This reminds us of the consumption of personal identity symbols.

There were many interview transcripts that could be analysed to support the suggestion that having a good and secure sense of *individuality* (the denoted emic meaning being about 'doing your own thing', and 'not worrying what others think') confers 'subjective power'. There is a familiarity in this notion that the individual can be central and disconnected to the forces around himself. All the transcripts emphasise and reinforce the notion that power is owned by people, like the contents of a saving account. In the sentiments 'most people think I'm a ward manager', Bob (see *Case 3*) is suggesting that this elevation in status and authority is, in part, due to his appearance as an older male nurse. He means that his persona tricks people into thinking he is something that he is not. Yet it is the expectation that older male nurses are more than likely to 'be in charge' or 'have the experience' necessary for being a ward manager that is identified by this type of incident. However, as already suggested using the semiotic analysis, it is a myth to believe that an individual or group is either totally powerful or completely powerless. The 'meaning' of power for Bob is the dominant model, a model based firmly on patriarchal order, hierarchy, and the individual. For Bob, it is his individual appearance, not his sex, that tricks people into assuming he has power; image (representation) not individuality. For male nurses, power is about meeting the needs of the organisation as well as the individual (subject) as suggested by James (*Case 3 Interviews*):

> '...oh yeah, the other difference is ordering people around isn't it ? To be honest most of the nurses I know don't do that, you know. I think it's because we all know what we're doing anyway, but there are some that think they own the place the way they tell you every little thing they want doing. They think because you're not trained that you haven't got a brain and that... that pisses me off you know. Being a bloke doesn't really come into it I don't think.'

For those who perceive themselves as having no organisational power, there is relief in the form of perceiving that they have 'inner power'; this is of symbolic importance. James, like many male non-trained nurses, talks about the *differences* that make them, as an occupational group, special and particular. He is good with patients, he does 'escorts', and 'the breakfasts'; in fact, the researcher was told he is a 'sound nurse to have in your team'. Yet the topic of power for junior nurses, as with managers, is fraught with attempts to denote logically sounding and plausible explanations of power dynamics: 'being the boss means that you have no choice, but to exercise power', or the rationale: 'non-trained staff have their own type of power, they are good with the patients and that's the most important thing'. However in this case, the connotations relate to lower grade nurses 'not being as good as trained nurses', that 'if they were more committed, they would have done their training', or 'perhaps it is just a career stepping stone', or 'are they just not capable?' The possibility that male nurses, like James, fulfil their role using agreed standards set down in cultural meaning is an uncomfortable proposition. The notion being that 'I am in change and control of my own world as an individual with identity and agency', 'that I choose the way I perform my signs', is one that provides a powerful nursing cultural myth for many male nurses, as they feel the full impact of maleness discourse on their subjective and subjected bodies.

One individual regardless of the 'the self' cannot exercise power that changes cultural meaning. For example, the nurses who spoke about 'just being themselves' and 'not letting anyone change the way they work' genuinely believed that their 'inner self' contributes to the already established culture, but what this study has brought to the fore is the way male nurses are unaware of maleness, and their inability to resist the representation of it in their cultures. For it is the representation of signs that has significance, not the 'inner self'. The folk terms, brought to the researcher, were those replications of expected cultural knowledge about what had meaning as being 'the best' in their culture. The self, therefore, seems to be just a vehicle. It enables the performance of sex role traits. We are reminded of the symbolic interactionist insistence that individuals interact in a dynamic and meaningful way, as opposed to (re)producing specific signs (Goffman, 1959). It is with this idea of (re)production that the discussion continues.

As James (*Case 3*) points out, money is an obvious pointer to hierarchy within nursing, but it is not the only one. The focal data used in this discussion suggests that people have power because they occupy certain roles; some fleeting and unnoticed, and some newly created within specific interactions. These roles allow each subject access to particular symbols of power. Nurses are also positioned in roles by language, rituals, tradition, and behaviour because different signs (ways of speaking and performing) are associated with such roles. The signs, as consumed and then performed by male nurses, are easily identified, (re)produced, and consumed by other nurses. The (re)production of sex role traits, such as a concern for power, hierarchy, and status, are those identified by the informants as being connected more to male nurses than to female nurses. Yet there continues to be an insistence that this denotes a 'truth', or as evidence that biological inheritance and genetic determinism, as opposed to social forces, is the cause.

This dominant myth indicates that psychiatric nursing cultural knowledge in the wards is somehow unable to be acknowledged, except in terms of specific performances of stereotypical male sex role traits. But it doesn't answer the question, What is it about the human condition that continuously propels us to enter power relationships and then, despite protests like that of James, perpetuate them? What is it about the connotations of these myths that nursing cultural knowledge is unable to acknowledge? Janet Hyde (1985), one of the first authors of a textbook on the psychology of women to include a chapter on the psychology of men, points out that there is now a 'self-aware psychology of men', rooted in feminism, and conscious of the power of gender roles, and particularly of how the male role influences the lives of men. Even so, the perceived power that individual male nurses seek is about 'keeping stumm', 'brown nosing', 'commitment' and 'blagging'; having an 'easy life', lack of 'involvement', specified and preferred types of 'ownership' and 'job security'. And, in *Case 3*:

'doing the job', 'carrying the responsibility', 'having a go', and 'taking the lead'. These are all included terms that informants use to describe the way 'perceived personal power' can be enacted, embodied, and be culturally useful. Such self-aware-ness is identified as a sense of *detached individuality*, and the notion of an engaging community—it shapes a tribe, a group of like-minded, 'naturally' occurring individuals who share similar attitudes.

Tribes

The decision to call this section 'Tribes' was a conscious one, because it is argued that, at an anthropological level, what makes tribes is cultural difference. Most anthropology is the search for the difference that makes a tribe unique. Thus, 'Tribes' as a section title brings us to the recurring notion of *binary oppositions*. It is a central semiotic theme and also one that dominates gender theory.

It has been argued, so far, that there is a massive differ-ence in the types of signs male nurses are expected to (Re)Pro-duce in their representations of maleness. In the face of much objection to this claim (the emic assumption being that there are a few differences, and that these are only due to biological determinants, and that all humans are individuals who have agency), this section will stress the significance of this theoreti-cal position in answering the previously posed question about what propels people into relationships of power? Part of the way of doing this made use of the (re)production theme, as a method for understanding cultural meaning (collecting folk terms, creating taxonomies, re-testing these, then asking the question, What do these domains tell me about the connota-tions of this culture?), and it has been possible to produce the domain, 'Power/hierarchy is used to do maleness'. Part of the cultural theme is also, *(Re)producing masculinity is the opposite of performing femininity and homosexuality, or not acting straight (binary opposites).*

The underlying feature of opposites has been frequently explored in feminist literature (Irigaray 1992; Kristeva, 1982; Derrida, 1976; Foucault, 1973) and it is argued that it is possi-ble to subject the concept of masculinity to the same type of post-feminist/post-structuralist semiotic analysis (identifying the connotation/identifying the dominant discourse/locating the episteme—the way knowledge is maintained/decentering the subject/deconstructing the grand narratives). This fragmenting of masculinity, as performed by both Connell (1987) and Mac an Ghaill (1994), is the key to understanding the different kinds of power masculine sub-types with their various symbols. This is particularly related to relations of alliance, dominance, and subordination. These relationships are constructed through practices that exclude and include, that intimidate, exploit, and so on. As just discussed, male nurses perform power in terms of symbols and signals for other men to recognise and 'consume'. Of central importance is the recognition of the obvious fragmentation of the male subjective across time and space. Masculinity, therefore, becomes masculinities (plural). Though patriarchy protects male power and authority, it does not protect all individual men equally and in the same way. Rather, it protects certain patterns of power and promotes those types of behaviour conducive to their preservation (Buchbinder, 1998).

Various ideological imperatives and myths (such as essentialism (myth 1), naturalism and truthful reality 'out there' (myth 2), gender difference is biological (myth 3), male nurses are more in touch with their feminine side (myth 4), and power belongs to individuals (myth 5)) help to constitute maleness, and they are, in turn, supported and ratified by it. Extending across the entire social structure, maleness seems to function rather like a class system. The tribes are segregated, some excluded or marginalised, those deemed too effeminate, dominant subjects, inferiorised subjects and 'the other' subjectivities, all define those subjectivities in the tribe that maleness defines as central. For example, during *Case 2*, one particular non-trained male nurse was the butt of most jokes (even in his presence). He was called an 'arse licker' and 'a brown nose', that he couldn't be 'relied on'. As an observer, the author concluded that he was being made an outcast, subjugated, inferiorised. The signs were obvious. He was not what Mac an Ghaill (1985) would describe as a 'macho lad'.

In this way, maleness seems to rank and, thus, creates power differentials even among those it puts at the centre of things. Buchbinder (1998) discusses the patriarchy that the author accepts as being similar to power in operation as he observed the tribe, and says: 'differences among individual men, such as age, physical size and strength, class, wealth, social or political clout, sexual activity or hyperactivity—even penis size, and so on, are inverted with varying degrees of patriarchal power' (p43). It is this type of investment that enables maleness to impact on the subject, the Connell (1987) hegemonic masculinities, the tribe and culture. Although Connell differentiates a number of types of masculinity, it perhaps needs to be stressed, as done by O'Donnell (1997), that he considers hegemonic masculinity has been successful in 're-butting the challenges to it'. Similar to this study, Connell (1995), in his work entitled *'Masculinities'*, uses four sets of case studies and concludes, in a fashion similar to Mac an Ghaill, that masculinity is an important area of study. Both writers do not pretend to quantify the 'importance' of various masculinities. Rather, in a similar way to this study, they provide a high level of empathic understanding.

The one implication of this that can be observed and induced from the interviews is the degree of conformity by subjects. Maleness determines the requirements and measurements to see if 'you're man enough'; to see if your performance warrants the removal of your power. Yet, ironically within the tribe (all of the boys together), it is non-conformity that is often overtly and explicitly offered as the ideologically loaded and valued sign of the masculine; remember the taxonomy of non-femaleness: 'showing off', 'not caring', 'independence', 'being demanding', 'not being boring'. The boyish dare, the mischievous gesture at the ward manager both lead to a subject knowing his place. To recognising, via auto-identification, his masquerade that he is something different away from work. All nurses are not equal regardless of the slogans of nursing discourse. To be 'top dog' is to be at 'the top of the tree'. A male nurse's status and power, and thus his identity and ability to perform, is dependent upon his ability to understand the knowledge of cultural signs. He needs to be able to perform these sign and represent the expected attributes of maleness.

Summary: Subjectivization by maleness

What has been argued up to this point? That maleness discourse (patriarchy and masculinity in psychiatric nursing culture) subjectivizes all nurses. It shapes the way in which the experience of subjects is perceived and given cultural 'meaning'. This meaning is made up of myths that denote meaning, but also always have ideological connotations, encouraging and discouraging nurses to see in certain ways, and not in others, and prompts the nurses to accept and emulate or to reject and condemn certain behaviours ((re)produced via signs) or attitudes.

The discourse, as can be seen from the similarity of folk terms that dominate the taxonomies of this study, determines who has the status, hierarchy, authority to speak about a topic or to whom. In addition, as noted by Buchbinder (1998), 'it determines where and when a topic be addressed' (p11). In this way, sites of status and power are established and maintained.

The issue of subjectivization is inferred and indicates that it is possible, and plausible, to identify ideological myths that support the idea of the existence of a maleness discourse. The existence of a nursing discourse is more readily accepted, whereas the former is often denied and, if acknowledged, only as 'non-different' between the natural and biological sexes. It is clear that several ideologies are encoded in the nursing discourse (the discourse of gender (maleness), the discourse of medicine, the discourse of humanism, etc). This coalescence of multiple ideologies allows, not only for variety, but for contradiction and conflict. This, in turn, indicates that power is distributed unequally through nursing culture. Maleness can be seen as a dissenting discourse, in which nurses are subjectivized to exercise positions of power, privilege, and status.

The discourse of nursing (in psychiatry) with its promotion of individualism, nurturing, caring, and patient-centred ideologies finds itself overshadowed by the imposing figure of patriarchy. When a male nurse enters into nursing discourse, he is subjectivized into the discourse of maleness. It impacts upon him. He is now a subject of maleness and will (re)produce its encoded symbols and myths, and the connotations they harbour. He will represent that which is framed within cultural knowledge; that a cultural knowledge is a form from which female nurses are not barred, because they are just as subjectivized. The impact of maleness on the subject affects the identity, performance, individuality, status, vulnerability, and power of all subjects.

It is with this impact on all subjects that the following sections of the discussion will focus. They will argue that the impact of maleness on nursing discourse is not so much a clash of the Titans, but rather a continuous process of abrasion/attrition of one discourse on the subject, one that is constituted in the cultural knowledge of signs, symbols, and difference. To do this the following sections examine symbolism, collective identity, and difference within psychiatric nursing culture.

It seems that male nurses perform, as often as possible, those traits perceived in terms of cultural knowledge, as having the best desired effect of legitimising their identity. The cause and effect relationship in the emic view is the opposite to that argued in this book. The emic view would be that male nurses naturally behave the way they do because they have an inner self, which is genetically masculine. They do things differently (i.e. reproduce masculinity) because they are male and because there is a social expectation, or social forces acting upon them. But they can resist these social forces, if they have a strong enough inner self. They can, therefore, choose how they behave. This is typically summed up by Simmy (*Case 3 Interviews*) who argues that power is within us all. We can draw upon it to achieve desired effects. It does not necessarily have anything to do with relationship structures.

> '...I don't think its about power really. I've had to deal with a lot of racial stuff, but I don't think its about power. I get all of my power from myself. If I want things to happen then I'm responsible for getting it done, aren't I?'

Chapter 7
Machismo, the manmade symbols

'Male aggression and lust are the energising factors in culture. They are men's tools of survival in the pagan vastness of female nature.'

Camille Paglia (1992)

'...I remember one time thinking that I could be sitting on the legs of my mom and wondering how she would like it?

James (Machoness)

Machoness is an attribute of maleness

This chapter focusses on the cover term 'machoness' in psychiatric nursing culture. Machoness, as an emic folk term, is perceived to be one of the most decisive gender traits (collection of signs) that represents 'difference' between male and female, and psychiatric and general nursing cultural knowledge. The assumptions made of machoness, as a process of representing maleness, is attributed to its reliance on stereotypes and symbolism. Even though the nurse informants assume that 'individuals' and their identity are either more or less macho, or that male nurses can chose if they want to be macho, how often and by how much, there is no acknowledgement that male nurses cannot stop representing maleness, or being judged upon their (re)production of its signs and symbolism. This chapter is the first to concentrate on the impact of maleness on the site of cultural knowledge. It extends the discussion by interpreting the myth (myth 6) that *there is a natural relationship between the signs and symbols of the 'out there reality' and their meaning* and, further, that there is a simple relationship of *reflection* between oneself and an objective, real, pre-existing, universal truthful world. The discussion progresses through the following points:

1. Psychiatric nursing cultural knowledge is exchanged using signs and symbols;

2. Signs and symbols are constituted by cultural knowledge;

3. Therefore, subjects are not responsible for the arbitrary meaning of the symbols they perform. Their meaning already exists and is just being (re)produced; and

4. To be a male nurse you are identified by your ability to (re)produce stereotypic behaviours.

The next three sections are concerned with how cultural knowledge in psychiatric nursing culture interprets the cover term and symbol (*connotations*) of machoness. It seems to be an inevitable burden of being a man. It is a collection of signs and a symbol that represent particular types of behaviour associated with men. The term is often derogatory when applied to women, as though they are non-sexual and, therefore, not a woman or a man. For men, the term has transformed itself over time from the 1960s, as portrayed in the Hollywood classics when every man wanted to be a Tarzan or Ben Hur, to become an embarrassment by the 1990s. In order to begin exploring it, these sections will provide the emic definitions, the informants' views. These views reflect the typical denotations about gold medallion wearing, bronze tanned men who flex their muscles in public. The sections will also continue to develop the thesis that it is not individual males who create machoness, but rather the cultural knowledge that is constituted by and constitutes the typical representations of machoness. Specific focal data will be put forward to support this theoretical position.

The following three sections emphasise the important issues of language, the representation of expected symbols and sexuality. The domain, 'Machoness is an attribute of maleness', allows for an examination of them in practice. Many of the accounts given by nurse informants emphasised the stereotypic, the difference, the expectations, and multi-faceted themes related to machoness as an attribute of maleness. Yet the issues of language, expected behaviour, and sexuality emerged as the most forceful. It is with these that the sub-themes emerged from the data. These provide a framework for arguing that maleness has an impact on nursing culture, but in an unexpected and objectionable way. It is often supposed that male nurses, as 'individuals', chose to do Maleness, yet the data interpreted by the researcher suggests that maleness does them.

The argument that has been unfolding throughout the previous chapters has introduced the idea that maleness has cultural meaning. Representation of it actually produces culture and not *vice versa*. This means that a sense of *identity*, shared knowledge, and language contributes to the production and consumption of meaning. Difference between male and female nurses exists, not primarily due to sex, but to the positioning of subjects within the representation of maleness and the (re)production of its meaning. Females represent the limit of maleness because the body is a status symbol.

The issue of power and hierarchy was identified as an icon of the supposed individuality and centeredness of the subject presumed to have agency. Yet it is not the individual who has agency, but the cultural myths that allows this impression. It is discourse—not things in themselves—that constitutes knowledge of what power is. Male nurses are not more powerful as subjects (than females—the other), rather, they are representing maleness, which is more powerful in power's circulation of competing discourses.

The discussion will continue the argument that, as subjects rather than individuals, male nurses are used to do maleness; that they use signs and symbols to represent maleness by (re)producing uses of language/behaviour and by acting straight rather than acting gay. More importantly, the issue of machoness enables us to explore the impact of maleness on men as they feel it; the '(re)production dread' they endure to represent that cultural knowledge, which is deemed acceptable. Because status and power impact on them, as they represent it, it seems that 'being macho' and proving your sexuality goes to the core of what male nurses perceive as their identity and performance of 'the self'.

Trapped in language: trapped in cultural knowledge

All signs are arbitrary—there is no natural relationship between the sign and its meaning or concept. Signs themselves cannot fix meaning. Meaning is relational. There is no simple relationship of reflection, imitation or one-to-one correspondence between language and the real world.

Myth (6) emphasises the importance of language in culture. In particular, it highlights the notion that all signs and symbols observed in psychiatric nursing culture have cultural meaning. Each sub-theme overlaps and is a contextual narrative as opposed to a definite truth. The introduction to the three sections will note the emic and dominant denotations given by nurses (see *Figure 7.1*).

● Work is a result of maleness	● 'Being late' is an attribute of maleness	● 'Cheek' is used to do maleness	● 'Promotion' is a way to do maleness
● 'Having attitude' is a result of Maleness	● 'Career building' is an attribute of maleness	● 'Self-respect' is used to do maleness	● 'Having knowledge' is a way to do maleness
● 'Having an easy life' is a result of maleness	● 'Being demanding is an attribute of maleness	● 'Self-esteem' is used to do maleness	● 'Being able to show your skills' is a way to do maleness
● Sticking together' is a result of maleness	● 'Not caring' is an attribute of maleness	● 'Enthusiasm' is used to do maleness	● 'Showing off' is a way to do maleness
● 'Paying the mortgage' is a result of maleness	● 'Tiredness' is an attribute of maleness	● 'Self-worth' is used to do maleness	● 'Being motivated' is a way to do maleness
● 'Being detached' is a result of maleness	● 'Job security' is an attribute of maleness	● 'Being away from home' is used to do maleness	● 'Money' is a way to do maleness
● 'Bad atmospheres' are a result of maleness	● 'Using your brain' is an attribute of maleness	● 'Avoidance' is used to do maleness	● 'Easy life' is a way to do maleness
● 'Unequal work load' is a result of maleness	● 'Being motivated' is an attribute of maleness	● 'Acting like a man' is used to do maleness	● 'Full time' is a way to do maleness
● 'Not being boring' is a result of maleness	● 'Having more confidence is an attribute of maleness	● 'Non-femaleness' is used to do maleness	● 'Looking towards the future' is a way to do maleness
● 'Management' is a result of maleness	● 'Being independent' is an attribute of maleness		● 'To provide for your family' is a way to do maleness
● 'Not having to worry about the children' is a result of maleness	● 'Being God's gift' is an attribute of maleness		

Figure 7.1: Preliminary domain analysis (maleness) in *Case 2*

When I tried to grab him I managed to just hold him so we could talk...I didn't have to do much more than that...I didn't do anything special, but everyone else seemed to think I was the main man.

How often does it happen for the men in your ward ?

It depends on the patients.

When a male nurse interacts with a distressed and potentially aggressive patient, as described in the extract above by James (*Case 3 Interviews*), what goes through his [the nurse's] mind? Is it the safety of the patient, colleagues or absolutely nothing? Is it an instinct reaction, or is it a conscious decision with strategic significance within his relationship with that patient? What are the results of dealing with an aggressive patient? Some of the included terms are 'safety', 'just doing your job', and 'working through difficult issues'. However, let's assume that James had not stood in the way of the aggressive patient. Let's assume that the patient was, indeed, aggressive and not just being loud, upset, and 'letting off steam'. Perhaps he **was** going to physically attack the other patient who was tormenting him. What would it mean if James had not been brave, been a hero, done what male nurses are supposed to do? When asked, James and other male nurses never consider this to be an option. They are trapped by their maleness and the *symbolism* of their performances.

The idea that the language we all use is neutral is a common one among the nurse informants in the case studies. It is assumed that individuals use language to express themselves as authentic authors and choose particular phrases in order to exchange information. Some language is thought to be more expected from male nurses, such as swearing and sexist jokes. In addition, the way that language is uttered is considered to share a relationship with the gender of the person speaking it. For example, during the field work it was observed that male nurses were louder and more expressive in their behaviour. There was a general assumption that this was to be expected because they were men. It would be perfectly possible for men and women to do the same thing, but for it to be labelled different. For females, this has been a constant point of discussion be it about women drinking from pint glasses or telling smutty jokes.

Being trapped in language, and in the expected symbols of behaviour, is a position posited by this thesis, yet it has little resemblance to how the nurse informants perceive their everyday practice. Apart from the discrimination just noted, most nurses might moan about 'unfairness' as if not being able to swear were a disadvantage. But, nevertheless, the hypothesis of 'being trapped' in the symbolism of the myth, even if there is no consciousness of the fact, is supported by the evidence adduced from this study.

For example, many of the nurses told stories about other male nurses who had a reputation for either 'sorting things out', or 'being unreliable when restraining aggressive patients'. Others talked about the 'sissy nurse' who couldn't take the pressure, or the 'solid charge nurse' who never went off sick. These men perform the symbols of maleness. They have to perform specific macho behaviours to create for themselves a niche in the cultural meaning of what it is to 'sort things out'. Connotations are reinforced and the young male staff nurse is pressured to aspire to be 'a solid charge nurse', thus, following the ritualistic structures and rites of passage. These structures are interwoven in the cultural meaning of what it is to be macho. To be 'solid', the male nurse has to be 'a good listener', 'be able to care', 'show his emotions', 'be firm, but fair', 'have nerves of steel', 'be a good laugh', and 'never forget his mates'. James knew what he had to do to represent the 'sound' male nurse performing behaviour, and this reflects the fact that language does not simply mirror gender. It helps constitute it—it is one of the means by which gender is enacted, symbolised and then consumed.

For the purpose of this extended argument, gender is not a noun, it is a verb. We do gender, we are doing gender every day in the wards in an attempt to (re)produce cultural meaning in terms of representing maleness in nursing. The following transcripts give a feeling that to fail in the 'act of machoness' is to fail maleness and, therefore, be the other; that is, something, which is not maleness, e.g. a female or homosexual.

> '...It's very rare that I get called to intervene with a female patient...I remember one time thinking that I could be sitting on

the legs of my mom and how would she like it ? But at the time it's important to work as a team and help her work through her anger.

'...We're all the same, male nurses just hang around the edges of any incident and let the females try and talk them down. It's only if things start to get out of hand we act. ...It's about the dignity of the patient, if she's cat fighting and that, the last thing you want to do is make it worse.'

(James; Case 3)

During *Case 1*, the author coined the phrase 'Male patients require male nurses'. This was a preliminary attempt to acknowledge that male nurses are seen as being employed to deal with aggressive patients. This notion is important to all male nurses in psychiatric nursing culture. They have no choice but to face it when an incident arises. To 'bottle it' is to symbolise a failed representation. As noted in the transcript, male nurses are expected to wait before restraining. This last resort process would be violated if a male nurse restrained a patient before talking to them; they would be viewed as breaking the cultural norm and 'doing bad practice'. Nursing discourse ideology determines that nurses 'use the self', that 'violence is not the answer' and emphasises 'dignity of the patient'. Likewise, to 'bottle it' is to produce signs that go to implode the identity of maleness. It seems that a male nurse, unlike female nurses, has to 'represent maleness' before everything else. Imagine the embarrassment of Bob (*Case 3 Interviews*) in the extract below:

'...One young lady received a clout around the ear. I felt really bad inside, thinking to myself that I should have stopped it from happening, but as always, these things are there for us to learn. Which I certainly did. The old charge nurse looked down at me as I pathetically tried to scrabble around with this patient. He was only a small lad like I said, but as slippery as an eel. ...I don't think I was flavour of the month with that female nurse.'

To represent maleness is to be trapped in language and behaviour. If a male nurse were able to chose, would he not seek alternative approaches? What about instinct, for example, the courageous soldier who throws himself on the grenade to save his platoon (Hollywood films are full of such heroism)? What about the argument, 'I do it because it feels right'? Maleness is about the cultural meanings that encase the male body. Maleness does production, subjects do consumption. Male nurses do machoness to save others, to be heroes, to be the best, to have an 'identity', to be modest 'individuals', to exercise 'a performance, a masquerade', to get promotion, and because it is something to do. What else can they do? Perform like female nurses? There is a constant argument that there are no differences between the sexes, but the impact of maleness produces difference. Sure enough, a female nurse can (re)produce machoness, she will be seen as aggressive and non-approachable. She will be viewed as being different in herself, or as being essentially different from that which she is expected to be, i.e. female. Male nurses are supposed to be naturally masculine. There is no naturalness about masculinity, it is a construct, and male nurses have no choice other than to be trapped in the representation (production), symbolism, and consumption of it. The following section demonstrates the difficulties associated with these performances that are grounded in cultural knowledge.

(Re)production dread

Nursing is inseparable from the relationship it has with this wider culture. Nursing has traditionally promoted the cultural myths prevalent in the wider culture of society of which it is part. Nursing discourse is about caring, helping, being feminine.

Once again, Bob (*Case 3 Interviews*) was able to describe an incident when he found himself wrestling with his own performance of machoness rather than a patient:

*'On other units I've not noticed that so much. I've certainly found myself…err…in a wrestling match and having to be **macho**. One incident, the first person to get to the unruly patient was a female colleague, a woman member of staff, she got the first tussle, and the bounding and then we all joined in. She was not in the least bit afraid. She didn't look round for a chap, she*

just got on with it. She said that sometimes there's not a bloke around and we can't have patients hurting each other. This happened on the **ITU** *so I guess she'd selected herself for that.'*

If male nurses are not trapped in the discourse of maleness, then they do not have to be concerned with the symbols of machoness or the representation of maleness. The demonstration that they would restrain patients simply because they were nurses, the same as their female colleagues, would suffice to justify that no difference existed, and that all individuals and their identities were unique and, therefore, probably unpredictable most of the time. However, the consistent message from interview data and observations strongly suggest that, even though performing machoness is, at times, a laughing matter, at others sexual, yet at other times it is an inclusion/exclusion criteria for male nurses who huddle together talking about the stereotypical topics of football, other sports, and playing golf. In a culture of maleness, rewards are always distant and at a premium. They must be fought over competitively; male nurses have to instantiate the sense of destiny—an awareness of the power conferred upon men by the world of work and money. A world full of folk terms, such as 'paying the mortgage', 'being away from the wife and kids', and 'being hard'. Thus, we enter the world of (re)production dread. A world which emphasises the need for male nurses to learn, copy, and complement the (re)production of social signs and uphold (via the myth) the representation of maleness. A world in which consumption drives production not *vice versa*. Yet, production is (re)production, a copy of the sign symbolised in cultural knowledge.

Ways	Results	Uses	Attributes
'don't be moody' 'practical jokes' non-'bitching' non-'gossiping' 'no need to compromise' 'so you don't keep hurt'	'more fun' 'have a laugh' 'arguing in public' 'feeling left out' 'keeping distanced' 'keep yourself to yourself' 'having control'	'letting people know that you are pissed off' 'letting out your anger' 'by getting all of the crappy jobs' 'always having to do the little jobs'	'not giving a shit' 'having an easy life' 'isolation from colleagues' 'defensiveness' 'by not getting too involved'

Figure 7.2: Taxonomic analysis for the preliminary included terms related to the semantic relationship: 'Is a result of maleness'

Ways	Results	Uses	Attributes
'not being too pushy' 'not being a house husband' 'missing the children' 'making money' 'building a career'	'to have a good life/working professional relationships'/'being a good role model'/'respect from others' 'confidence'	'make sure you're busy'/'have planned activities'/'go off the ward' 'do jobs badly the first time so that you're not asked again'	'being true to yourself'/'earning it'/'doing a good job'/'recognition'

Figure 7.3: Taxonomic analysis for the preliminary included terms related to the semantic relationship: 'Is used to do maleness'

Ways	Results	Uses	Attributes
not being part-time being sensible not wearing yourself out being lazy singing in the day room juggling tots	flexibility more money having fun being a prat making the day go quick getting attention	get better jobs 'getting a bad name' 'doing bank' 'doing agency' 'doing two jobs' 'trying to be important' 'showing people that you're good at something'	'planning a career' 'keeping your eyes open for other jobs and promotion' having respect for other men

Figure 7.4: Taxonomic analysis for the preliminary included terms related to the semantic relationship: 'Is a way to do maleness'

The intrinsic difficulty with the sex-role theory is how it consistently implies that there can be a 'self' for the individual outside the sex role; that we, as individuals, acquire or learn the sex role on top, as it were, of our own identities or sense of self. The expressions given in the figures above demonstrate this obsession with 'the self'. It may be thought that, by removing the sex roles and the necessity to (re)produce the attributes of these roles, a real 'self' can be released from underneath. This self can, in a traditional humanistic way, grow and reach its full potential independent of a sex role. However, this social and philosophical idealism, which would supplant sex roles with other roles, begins to look very much like social engineering and attempts to universalise the supposed nature of the individual. Male nurses are products of their culture. It is the cultural knowledge they (re)produce as subjects.

Nursing culture is a culture that proposes the symbolism of 'soft masculinity'. Yet it is masculinity all the same. The idea must be that no individual can be stripped of what is fundamentally their basic identity. No cultural subject can be thought of as not having a 'self' underneath their sex role. Having mentioned that, recognition is the first important step; it is followed by trying to understand how a male nurse learns to define himself, and others, within an environment that he must negotiate constantly. There are also rites of passage 'on becoming a male nurse'. A painful, but seemingly inescapable rite, is the psychiatric nurse's loss of innocence—the dread of failure—of not being accepted, of failing to (re)produce the symbolism of maleness to a 'meaningful' standard (some of which are given in *Figure 7.5*); of replicating the great feats of charge nurses, since promoted, compound the dread that male nurses face.

The nostalgic vision of male-centred rituals (partly recoverable from myths, stories, and the practices of other nurses) serves to remind nurses of the expectations placed upon them. Yet the constant references to the identity, individual, and personal traits associated with performance of the self remind us that nursing cultural knowledge has discourses impacting upon it. From this, it would be argued by Baudrillard (1994), nursing consumes, and nothing is more obvious than the issue of sexuality.

Straight acting

If a male nurse is confident enough to be different, behave non-macho, perhaps be effeminate, then this is seen to be (re)producing something that is not masculine, or at least measurable against masculinity. There has been much gossip in nursing circles concerning the sexual orientation of male general nurses and of their supposed 'effeminacy'. This highlights the way the dominant patriarchal and homophobic culture

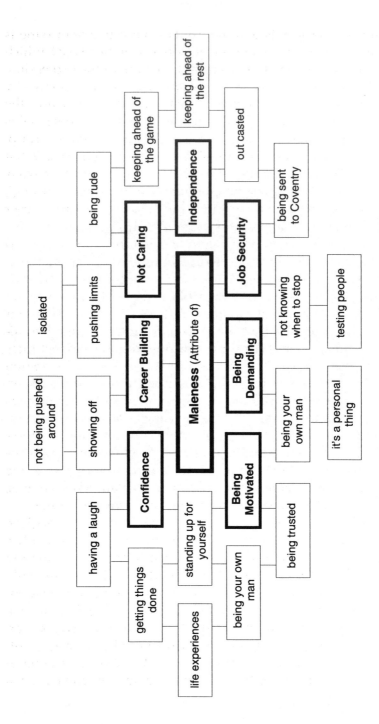

Figure 7.5: Template 1 Case 2): Significant included terms: 'is an attribute of maleness

attempts to secure its dominance. The discourse of nursing is asexual. Sexuality is a hang-over from times, since past, which place a cumbersome burden round the neck of the profession. The nurse informants in the case studies articulate politically correct (and probably insincere) assumptions regarding the sexuality of colleagues and themselves. To be heterosexual is to belong to the dominant, the normal, and the safest group. The ideologically loaded response to questions, such as, 'What are all the ways being effeminate ?' and 'What are all the ways male nurses are considered gay?' will include 'Nothing', 'None at all', 'It's not true', and [typically] 'It doesn't matter what orientation a person is as long as they're a good nurse'.

As expected, this type of response typifies the caring and understanding nature we have all become more accustomed to during the past twenty years. Yet the sniggers and laughs about 'being a shirt lifter' or 'not turning your back' remain the common phrases offered by males who retained their sense of sexual identity and attempt to protect it as the domi-nant discourse. The cultural meaning in the case studies emphasised a particular cultural theme, one that rests upon the assumption (as expected) of difference. Sexuality as an identity can represent the logical, in control, and machoness, and is represented by heterosexuality. The (re)production dread theme relates to the inability of a male nurse to repre-sent maleness (which is always heterosexual) by means of rit-uals, myths, soft masculinity, and the many other sex role attributes within cultural knowledge. To be an 'other', that is, to exemplify non maleness, is viewed as having a stigma.

To distance the feminine from the masculine, and achieve a subordination of the feminine (and hence also of women), is a cultural theme that includes sexuality. Psychiatric nursing culture is an environment that is conditioned to be sexually non offensive. Thus, 'straight acting' is a result of the sex-gen-der system that has cultural meaning. It is a performance, a masquerade of subjective identity with set scripts and prompts. When a male nurse is confronted with a gay col-league, he will act and convince himself that he is not homo-phobic. As an 'individual', he has made this choice. At a different level, the culture has become more tolerant, yet the 'hidden' discourse remains one of reluctant acceptance.

'Straight acting' implies that the doing of a kind of masculinity is also performing, as introduced in previous sections. The work of Goffman (1959; 1963) is relevant in his insistence of promoting the sex role models and performances of the self. Even if male nurses act and practise their performance, the discourse ensures that every man perform the conventional signs of masculinity in his body language, including aggressiveness, so as not to be stigmatised because of sexual orientation. We are also reminded of the vulnerability and performance anxiety, the unstable nature of the sign; the simulation that constitutes reality. Machoness in nursing is a good example to show how nursing culture no longer copies the real, but (re)produces it. Nursing discourse is an effect of wider representations where there is, seemingly, no dialogue between the symbolism and reality, only the signifying practices (performances).

The data from this study supports the view that psychiatric nursing culture, in terms of myths and its impacting discourses, naturalises and seduces nurses to believe that, as individuals, each nurse is unique. Individuals come to think in a particular range of ways, and to think a particular range of things. Nurses are subjected to many differing points of power, performance expectations, and an unstable sense of a reality 'out there'. This exposes a view that the way s/he perceives things is normal, natural, and universal. As members of a culture, they are subject to forces that are largely invisible and silent. These forces continually invite or order them to represent and display correct cultural signs. Thus, representation of the normal everyday things helps subjects to imagine themselves as 'self-fashioned and fashioning through identification of a particular set of traits or behaviours' (Buchbinder, 1998). This creates a feeling of authenticity when we, as subjects, are successfully interpellated by a particular (and especially ideologically approved) representation, such as nursing discourse.

Male nurses are conditioned by a (re)productive dread to conceal and suppress elements that might betray them to others as being insufficiently manly, or perhaps, insufficiently feminine. Even though male nurses perceive their reality as being one in which they are 'who they are' rather than just 'acting or performing', which has cultural meaning, the actual cultural theme identified by this study is just the reverse.

Chapter 8
The connotations of bricks and mortar

'A TOTAL institution may be defined as a place of residence and work where a large number of like-situated individuals, cut off from the wider society for an appreciable period of time, together lead an enclosed, formally administered round of life.'

Erving Goffman (1961, p1)

'I'm not sure if boundaries and routines are the same thing technically, but they do have the same role.... they both structure the day and that...'

Ally; Male Nurse

Institutions are a result of maleness

Institutions are not defined, as in the Goffman (1961) sense, as 'a place of residence and work', but rather, as webs of relationships, groupings, and pockets of *'collective identity'*, usually represented in the connotations of folk terms: 'all male nurses are the same', 'to be a male nurse you have to [behave] this way'. These are connotations because they are stereotypic and believed by the informants to be 'just generalisations'. Yet, not only does this way of speaking emphasise difference due to biological foundations, but it also operationalises the boundaries of how to be and not be a male nurse (perform and masquerade the valued and consumable signs). Being male is assumed to provide an *unchanging meaning and truth* (myth 7) and acts as a yardstick from which *all objectivity and subjectivity can be compared* and understood (myth 8).

1. Nursing cultural knowledge is perceived to be founded on a 'true' reflection of reality;

2. Having a sense of reality is synonymous with 'truth' and authenticity;

3. Yet, nursing culture is saturated with representations of what is 'best practice'. This saturation includes representations of wider society;

4. Therefore, the belief that signs function to represent an authentic realm of existence is self referential and a simulation; and

5. As an analytic theme, the idea of simulation remains poorly analysed, but is worthy of note due to its relation to the subjectivization of male nurses and cultural knowledge.

This section continues where the last chapter left off. It has the specific focus on nursing, as an institution that is a simulated collection of cultural myths. In the following chapters, two myths will be interpreted. First, (myth 7) *meaning and truth is unchanging because there is a constant reality 'out there' that can be objectively engaged with* and, second, (myth 8) that this constant and consistent reality *is objectively true and a yardstick from which all objectivity and subjectivity can be compared and understood.* To interpret these two myths, it will be asserted that nursing cultural knowledge becomes so saturated with representation that nursing experience can only take place at a removed level?

'Jobs for the boys'

Simulating collective identity

The subjectivization of each nurse means that they experience the culture they practice through a filter of preconceptions and expectations, fabricated elsewhere in advance. This fabrication and consumption of myth 'privileges image' above all other signs in the culture (Baudrillard, 1994). 'Jobs for the boys' is a well-known expression that has a broad 'meaning', related to how men club and stick together to protect the interest of men. At a semiotic level, the connotation is one of men taking care of men in terms of promoting friends and 'covering up'. It has a Masonic feel, but one that is often used to explain why certain male nurses are in the position they are. 'It's not what you know, but who you know' is a common expression, but, is it [true]? Does it have (re)production and consumption value for male nurses?

The development of the theme, 'Jobs for the boys', was induced from a number of other sub-themes that, at first, did not appear directly related to one another. The issues related to power, hierarchy, loyalty, companionship, and many other folk terms shared a common cover term. The male informants all acknowledged a certain type of 'difference' between the nature of their relationships with female colleagues compared to male colleagues. Some talked about a sex/friendship issue, some noted the need to keep up appearances, and others the need to 'just have a laugh' with their male colleagues.

The nurses in the case studies all prescribe to the myth that their world is a truthful and a direct reflection of empirically-based experience, gleaned through the five senses. Their world is 'out there'; it is something distinct and separate from the 'individual' who has an inner essence, an inner core. So how can this thesis put forward the idea that nursing cultural knowledge is a *simulation*? What evidence is there to suggest that the folk terms and collected taxonomies reflect the fake, the counterfeit, the second-hand, and the inauthentic?

The image of 'Jobs for the Boys' is just one of many taxonomies showing the way male nurses, collectively, protect the ideologies that come into contact with the individual (inner core-conscious level). These reactions are real; they effect, they cause, they are subjective experience and true. This is not denied. However, simulation should not be thought of as the opposite of truth. Simulation and reality seem to have a necessary attachment to each other.

The emergence of 'Jobs for the boys' as a cultural theme, almost as though it were an original phenomena of nursing reality, inspired the researcher to examine the relationship this cultural knowledge shared with subjectivization as a theoretical proposition. This examination progressed to the conclusion that there is no truth or falsity of representation, as there is with (re)production. What we have is a 'centreless' network of cultural knowledge that privileges the realm of representation. The belief that signs function to represent a fundamental authentic realm of existence remains the dominant model, one in which good nursing practice is perceived to be based in reality (as opposed to a simulation and just short of reality). Yet simulation is not just a copy. It is the real, because symbolism and representation is firmly embedded in the working lives of all nurse subjects. What this amounts to is that the reality of nursing culture is already simulated. It reflects the patriarchal networks outside of the institution, that is, male nurses (re)produce male images. And since reality is already simulated and motivated by consumption, they can only refer to simulation and not to some pure unadulterated reality.

Nurses desperately try to get out of simulation by producing events, activities, images, and representations that assure them of their reality. The male nurse will represent that which has cultural knowledge as being real and authentic, such as the typical male behaviour of 'playing the fool' and adhering to 'jobs for the boys' in a culture that is, according to Hicks (1996), 'archetypally feminine'.

Most of the male informants indicated that being a male nurse brought with it a type of representation of 'having a laugh'. This representation is something particular to male nurses, as opposed to female nurses and, therefore, signifies a *difference* between the performance of masculinity and that which is signified as 'proper' nursing. So, what is this 'having a laugh and why do male nurses represent masculinity in nursing in this way? The answer to these two questions will now be explored. It seems that male nurses recognise a particular (re)production of masculinity, symbolised in the way that they 'play the fool'; a sign that is simulated from what we know is funny or symbolic to 'having a laugh'. For example, 'always smiling', 'cracking jokes', 'pulling funny faces', and 'doing funny walks'. These signs are replicas we all know and recognise from our childhood; the peek-a-boo games, the irony and satire of the sit com. We think it is funny; we experience it as easy going and believe our experience to be based in a true reality. Yet cultural knowledge dictates what representations, what symbols (with their slippery signifiers) are funny.

Both female and male nurses like to have a 'fun' and relaxed working environment; what is different between the two groups is the way male nurses are marked against the yard stick of simulated representation, and expected to be happy-go-lucky, as described by Pat (*Case 3 Interviews*):

> *'Patients like it when men are around because we sort of entertain them...I think that we're fun and we show it. I know that the women do the same, but even they like to have fun. It makes for good practice. We do it naturally...*

The myth that 'having a laugh' is a job for the boys and is, therefore, a *natural* state of affairs, highlights the ideological assumptions that there definitely is *difference* between the two sexes, by the way they go about their daily nursing tasks. As noted by Ohlen and Kerstin (1998), 'there is a clear tendency to stress the importance of the identity of the nurse', which is about differences [between the sexes] in approaches to caring. Yet, there remains a need to promote theoretical clarity. To act like a fool is legitimised by the very myth that male nurses 'naturally' behave in this manner. In fact, if any male nurse does not act in this way, he is usually considered different himself, or 'moody'. This notion of what is natural and what is not (i.e. nurtured) seems to provide a type of stability rather than instability. A short extract by James (*Case 3 Interviews*) shows that he tries to get on with everyone by 'having a laugh'. He also highlights the belief that you have to know the rules in order to get away with it:

> *'...I think that everyone likes me here. I've been here almost a year now and I fit in, you know. It's all right. I have a laugh with the female staff...There's only one or two that you have to be careful with, but I know that it's the same wherever you go isn't it? I think that if I had to give a definitive answer, I'd say I try to get on with everyone whether they're male or female.'*

Not all male nurses openly admit that they 'play the fool'. Their professional conscience prevents them from considering that such a phenomena has any place in nursing. Such behaviour is marginalised, as belonging to those who do not shore up the standards of professionalism. Sometimes, the notion of 'the good old days' brings up pranks and laughs that nurses had in times gone by, but 'things are different now'. Now, a good nurse can use humour as a therapeutic skill, as a tool to improve patient care. This is the general defence of masculine foolery. But to be a good fool, a male nurse has to have reference to that foolery, which is known about and considered to be funny. The typical representations are those already in existence on TV and in the media. The representation of these symbols demonstrates a knowledge by the subjected fool and those who *consume* the signs. Nurses told of how they like to work in an environment that is fun and not miserable. The male fool simulates what is considered by the informants to be an objectively true reality, as an example of how liberated psychiatric nursing culture is.

The issue brings us to a questioning of what is valued in psychiatric nursing culture. All the themes and folk terms listed throughout this thesis can be seen as icons of what is valued in nursing culture. The simulation of *value* and *commodity use* is, indeed, a reflection of the reality 'out there', which is symbol saturated and, therefore, not truly reality in the mythical, natural sense. The value of symbols arises from particular interests. Nursing ascribes value to a cultural practice as a reflection of wider myths in society at large. Distinctions about what is valuable in nursing, as a collective identity, are generated by learned patterns of cultural consumption, which are internalised as being natural and, therefore, reality-based. To accept whole-heartedly the myth of reality 'out there' is to accept the consumer need of nursing as a collective identity. *Nursing cultural knowledge is driven to consume those simulated signs, which have value, and hold them up as useful representations of what nursing is about.* The male nurse who is easy to get on with is good. The whining, miserable male nurse is not good. Yet, it would be easy to miss the point that such moral judgements hide the myth that a truthful reality provides the benchmark, by which all of nursing culture, as an institution, is graded.

What this chapter has brought to the discussion is the argument that all signs and symbols are simulations of wider meaning, and that all signs have slippery signifiers that change over time. This means that the possibility of an objective, truthful reality can be questioned. Yet it is against this sense of truthful reality that nursing knowledge compares itself. This means that the value of representations is firmly based within the remit of powerful discourses and myths promoting those who sustain them. For maleness, this is about rendering the male subject a collective identity that has specific boundaries. Within these boundaries, each male nurse is expected to represent certain traits because they are mythically naturalised.

Chapter 9
We are what we are not

'Why is 'difference' so compelling a theme, so contested an area of representation? What is the secret fascination of 'otherness' and why is popular representation so frequently drawn to it?'

Stuart Hall (1997: 225)

'Men and to some extent women aren't allowed to be what they are because it's seen as being inappropriate for nursing'.

Leon (Male Nurse)

Non-femaleness is used to do maleness

The cultural meaning of what it is **not** to be a male nurse, has a direct relationship to what it **is** to be a male nurse. No construct is possible without 'an other'. This realisation draws us into the world of binary opposites, where people are searching for a sense of social identity and maintaining the arduous task of identity work. For male nurses, this work principally involves maintaining a distinct identity that is comparable to other men, and a performance and masquerade that is different from femininity. This is, according to Buchbinder (1998), because the female is one half of a binary discourse of 'transgressive homosexuality versus *normative* heterosexuality'. The myth of a metaphysical-centred individual, as autonomous, essential and universal, has resulted in the emic assumptions provided by the informants of this study. The binary discourse of difference is a *foundational* narrative myth in nursing, which is not only constituted in the wider discourse of patriarchal society, but also maleness. Myth (9) contends that *there are naturally occurring traits, which ensure that nursing is better suited for females, such as nurturing, caring, and being sensitive.* This section explores these issues, using focal data taken from the study.

1. Male performance is defined by what it is not, as well as by what it is;

99

2.   The symbols of maleness are those defining the boundaries;

3.   Non-femaleness is a collection of symbols that make use of the contrast principle in order to signify maleness;

4.   Nurturing, caring, and nursing are symbols of femininity; and

5.   These symbols form part of a myth that persists.

Nursing has traditionally been considered a female occupation, because females have the 'natural traits' of nurturing, caring, and motherliness. This typical and all-too-frequent myth (myth 9) provides the boundary of what it is to be a male nurse. It also reinforces, what Connell (1987) terms, 'emphasised femininity'. It is possible to examine this myth and interpret the way that male nurses attempt to represent masculinity, as nurturing, caring, and sensitive, by being something different, something masculine, and in opposition to femininity. As with all of the ethnographic themes provided in this discussion, the researcher synthesised current literature and found that it offers many facades to one theme: the theme of *difference*. The notion of representing 'non-femaleness' is not only the boundary of performing maleness, it is also the boundary of the study and thesis and, as such, brings us full circle to the start of the book.

The theme of 'non-femaleness' was introduced during *Case 2*. Nurses would refer to the 'difference', that is, the opposite sex, to help them understand and secure their own identity. The author began to think that one could not be substantiated without the other. Current post-feminist literature confirmed this interest 'in the other', and the theme was deemed worthy of discussion. This section is by no means given as a finale; it is not more or less important than the preceding sections. Instead, it is the shortest discussion section with the aim of describing the interdependence maleness maintains with non-femaleness in nursing cultural knowledge.

There is no maleness without non-femaleness

What are some of the things that male nurses do that are just a little bit feminine? The answer depends on the power and knowledge that the culture holds. As a cultural theme, the issue of non-femaleness is, itself, a binary opposition in opposition to the whole theme of this book—maleness. Femininity and masculinity, in terms of modernist logic, share a particular dialectical relationship. The assumption is that, where masculinity finishes, femininity begins (usually in that order). The responses to questions informants were asked, usually included some reference to femininity, as though masculinity and it representation could not exist without it, and in this respect, the informants were unanimous.

Although this section has only one theme, the theme of *difference,* it will be looked at in two ways. The first revisits the notion of *simulation* and introduces the idea of *masquerade* as something similar to 'acting straight' (Buchbinder, 1998); that is, a prepared performance, which maintains the norms of masculinity, not to secure the individual identity of men, but of maleness. This leads to the second notion of surveillance of *difference,* as a method of auto-identification and control (Foucault, 1980); that is, without a boundary or limit of representation, nursing knowledge could not make sense for the informants.

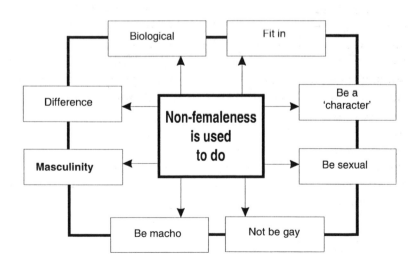

Figure 9.1: Non-femaleness is used to do maleness

Difference: Simulation and mas(queer)ade

Binary oppositions and difference hold a particular space in contemporary post-feminist and cultural studies. Similarities unite, difference categorises and, as discussed during the last section, these types of constructs are products of simulation, as shown in the opposed images of man-woman, Adam-Eve, hunter-gatherer, male nurse (psychiatry)-female nurse (general), and so on. This simulation of unquestioned essences has been politically dangerous for feminism and the male nurse, because the *connotation*, the secondary position of femininity, is often cited as being natural. This naturalness has had damning consequences for the 'hand maiden' found in nursing discourse; she, of course, is subservient to the patriarchal profession of medicine. There has always been a conscious effort to encourage more men into nursing in order to help raise its status (Lynn *et al*, 1975). Yet there remains an ambivalence towards the benefit of this for the profession. The primary *denotation* of the myth is to promote the improvement of patient care by increasing the **diversity** of skilled practitioners.

Nurses stressed this denotation of the myth. They constructed meanings for the researcher that had deliberate reference to *difference* as being necessary, natural, and beneficial to patient care. When asked, 'What are the main differences between the sexes in nursing?' the taxonomies quickly filled with reference to stereotypic (biologically determined) trait representations and cultural expectations made of the two sexes. Some of these included the traditional reference to 'logical masculinity' and 'sensitive femininity' Connell (1987). This type of yin-yang balance was viewed as being the harmony on which nursing culture operated, indeed co-operated and succeeded, to ensure that nurses of both sexes could secure an *identity*, a series of expected *performances*, be *individual*, maintain the *collective identity*, make sense of cultural *symbolism*, and respect *difference*.

In practice, however, the field work quickly enabled the researcher to realise that such harmony was multi-faceted and a simulation of nursing's attempt to replicate, consume and, therefore, simulate the cultural knowledge of the wider discourses from outside of the institution. In particular, the use of Thwaits *et al* (1994) enabled the researcher to conclude that, as subjects of a maleness discourse, the nurses in the psychiatric cultures were masquerading as the symbols expected of this wider discourse. The cultural knowledge of psychiatric nursing culture ensures that all knowledge is destined to reappear as simulation. Remembering that simulation anxiety creates an overwhelming desire in us all to hold onto nostalgia, to the natural, to the big wide world out there, it is not surprising that the informants cling to the sense of safety that their (sex type) gender identity seductively gives them. The father/mother archetypes, the buxom comforter, the sensible understanding uncle all comprise the masquerade of psychoanalytical persuasion, the Real English Men (Mac an Ghaill, 1985), the emphasised femininity (Connell, 1987), and the 'work role' (Tolson, 1977) that the nurses perform to reinforce the limits of *difference*.

The thesis is that maleness and nursing discourse constitute the nursing subject in simulating and masquerading the limits of their own gender identity. The emic view that they have a choice, an ability to 'add' particular appearances and subtleties on a natural and essential individuality (as argued by both Connell, (1987) and Weeks, (1985)), can be thought about as simulation (Baudrillard, 1994). So what about the emic view that difference created by maleness does not have an impact in nursing culture? The typical view told by informants is that 'all nurses are the same'. Some will note that male nurses are useful when patients are aggressive etc., [defending a role], but the general myth is one that has banished the ugliness of gender difference to the safety of the fringes, so that the female-dominated profession can be distanced from a perceived patriarchal take-over. However, any change in the definition of the feminine or the homosexual can induce a state of crisis in the masculine (Buchbinder, 1998). In the following extract Bob (*Case 3 Interviews*) once again intimates that the relationship between the two constructs is finely balanced:

'We're supposed to get stuck in when necessary, but surely isn't that just a reflection on what men are supposed to do or be like? I think, I've got the impression that, on this unit, the women collectively have a very strong recollection of when one of their colleagues was seriously hurt. She was a woman attacked by a male patient.'

Feminised in the eyes of his fellow nurses, the unfortunate male not only becomes more easily deprived of the signs of power, he may also become the butt of scorn, ridicule and sometimes aggression. Image and masquerade of parody is not tolerated in psychiatric nursing culture. There seems to be too much to lose for both maleness and nursing discourse. A male nurse who is too different, a female nurse who masquerades as too butch, will be marginalised. That is because they have a choice; they can either simulate the correct masquerade or face the consequences. What choice is that? It is a subjectivized choice.

Because of the competitiveness encoded in patriarchal discourse, myths and simulation, and the latter's resultant capacity to reward or penalise, in this culture men punish men for being men; but they also punish them for not being man enough. Male nurses are goaded to behave in a chivalrous way and believe stereotypically; perhaps they comply, not from some innate interest in protecting others, but rather to protect their own personal sense of self and, also, the stereotypic performance of masculinity in nursing as a collective. So, as male nurses, what are the expectations placed on them? This question was asked repeatedly. Below Simmy (*Case 3 Interviews*) ponders on this question:

'When I was doing my stint in general nursing, which in those days was three months, I noticed that there was a real marked difference between male and female nurses...ummm...well I mean, for instance I was called [Mr Smith]...females in my group were called nurse...These days...I'm trying to think about what the distinctions are between them...'

But nursing has always been done by women, so surely it is the male who should occupy a secondary position? First, men have been nursing as long as women; the modern preoccupation with the adventures of Florence Nightingale is a typical example of the history of key figures mystifying and distorting the relevance of discourse. Secondly, nursing discourse (as previously argued) cannot be separated from the wider culture in which it is situated. Nursing is constituted by the dominant ideologies prevalent in society. Therefore, it comes under the patriarchal medical discourse. Such patriarchal masculinity derives much of its power from a particular type of modernist logic. By imposing upon the flux of events a system of opposites, e.g., male/female, that logic not only produces meaning through difference, but equally gives those differences certain moral or ethical values, i.e. nursing is for women. As noted by Connell (1987), the idea that men are rational and women emotional has long been a theme in patriarchal ideology, one that continues to be consumed.

The performative identification of masquerade can either be employed to establish heterosexuality as compulsory, or to reveal its fictitious nature (Butler, 1990). It is the former compulsion that nursing and maleness discourse reinforces. Masquerade can either preserve or subvert the norms of a cultural knowledge.

Simmy (*Case 3 Interviews*) was asked the following question: [Well, what I'm interested in finding out is what are all the different kinds of male role?]

> '*Oh…well in my role I have to act as a good role model, that is, a good male role model because the patients need to learn from this…I think on the whole though, generally most male nurses that I've met try to nurse in a professional manner regardless of sex.*
>
> *I mean most male roles are those seen as strong and determined, but I've met lots of female nurses who are just the same really.*'

For Simmy, the meaning of 'the male role' should have nothing to do with sex, but he notes it has connotations regarding sexuality. It seems that the common protection for male nurses asked to confront sex and sexuality as a pre-determinant for how males are viewed (e.g. sexual animals), is the idea of professionalism. This identification can only take place due to 'auto-identification', i.e., when a person can acknowledge 'the other'. It is not professional to flirt or talk about sex with patients, particularly females. Simmy also argues that, apart from the 'sex and professionalism' issue, there is the notion that male roles promote a sense of order, but he is quick to say that it is the same for female nurses. This need to equalise difference in terms of professional issues in nursing is one that captures the whole essence of stereotypes and their meaning for male nurses. For many of the male informants, including Simmy, the issues of aggression, boundaries (and being able to work within them) and sexual urges are dominant facets in self-identification. Male nurses are very quick to understand the dangers of appearing either too oppositional, or too much in favour of these three so called typical traits, traits that are kept in check by professional boundaries.

Apart from the issue of professionalism, the meaning of typical male stereotypic behaviour is thought to harbour a 'naturalness'. To represent masculinity, male nurses have to be able to consume masculinity, which is assumed to be a natural phenomena. Boys will be boys and girls will be girls due to which biological sex they are. As an ideological construct, the performance of masculinity has similarities with a sense of naturalness within the commonsense boundaries of professionalism. Male nurses are allowed to represent masculinity because it is assumed that they have no choice. This is what can be called the 'simplified masculinity'—the stereotypic view of what it is to be a man—yet other masculinities exist that enlarge and partly contradict this mainstream stereotype. These other 'masculinities' (e.g. those identified by Connell (1987)), subordinated masculinity, complicit masculinity, marginalised masculinity, and those by Mac an Ghaill (1985): The Macho Lads, The Academic Achievers, and The Real English Men), once they are acknowledged, share a didactic relationship with the mainstream patriarchy that dominates the wards. These 'significant other' masculinities are becoming more widespread and unsettling to the considered norm (a natural, sexual, aggressive, order-maintaining, and professional masculinity). This makes the issue of self-identification and the meaning of maleness more diverse, fragmented, and perhaps a little more unsettling (crisis of masculinity).

Auto-identification requires the male nurse to identify a particular configuration of signs as, first, signifying 'masculinity' and, secondly, 'the other' (femininity) (Buchbinder, 1998). He is subjectivized as an ideologically obedient male subject who, as a performer, masquerades male performances that he recognises as being true to himself. This sense of authenticity is part of the process of auto-identification. Through a process of surveillance, the subject is able to identify himself. On the one hand, sexuality has everything to do with this identification, e.g. heterosexual and not being gay, but on the other, there is the idea that the simulation of nursing does not tolerate sexuality that uses masquerade as a means to nurse. This meaning can be inferred from all of the extracts given so far in this book. Some informants mentioned a final dominant meaning that has a relationship with stereotypic male behaviour: 'trying to get on'. Male nurses identify themselves in terms of 'the other', and perform masquerades of a competitive co-operation having a specific meaning for them as a collective.

Although nursing takes from the wider culture, its symbols and ideologies are such that they enable male nurses to perform within a masculine discourse, which dictates a feminine discourse. Yet it is this exposure that goes to define maleness.

The shared need to ensure that, as a male, you are not judged to be a woman is very important. Some of the male informants spoke of their friends and relatives being shocked and surprised when they started their nurse training. Others spoke about being proud to be psychiatric nurses, rather than general nurses. The implication seems to be that male general nurses are 'gay' and that psychiatric nurses have to wrestle with patients on a daily basis. This sense of difference is more profound in nursing than in any other setting. Therefore, the issues of masquerading and auto-identification serve to distance and legitimise obvious difference between the sexes. Male nurses reinforce the difference that nursing discourse attempts to hide. They do this because of maleness; they are

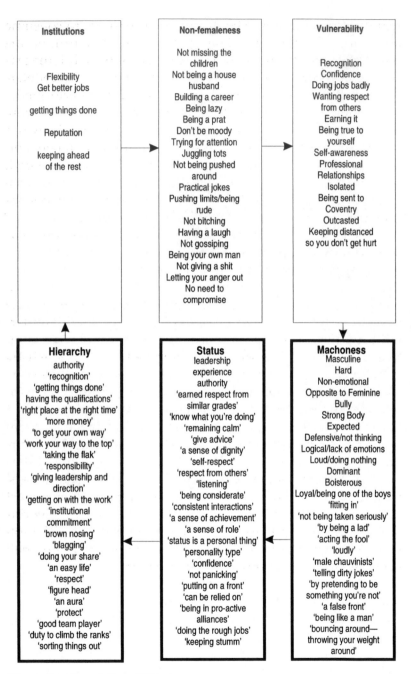

Institutions

Flexibility
Get better jobs

getting things done

Reputation

keeping ahead
of the rest

Non-femaleness

Not missing the
children
Not being a house
husband
Building a career
Being lazy
Being a prat
Don't be moody
Trying for attention
Juggling tots
Not being pushed
around
Practical jokes
Pushing limits/being
rude
Not bitching
Having a laugh
Not gossiping
Being your own man
Not giving a shit
Letting your anger out
No need to
compromise

Vulnerability

Recognition
Confidence
Doing jobs badly
Wanting respect
from others
Earning it
Being true to
yourself
Self-awareness
Professional
Relationships
Isolated
Being sent to
Coventry
Outcasted
Keeping distanced
so you don't get hurt

Hierarchy
authority
'recognition'
'getting things done'
having the qualifications'
'right place at the right time'
'more money'
'to get your own way'
'work your way to the top'
'taking the flak'
'responsibility'
'giving leadership and
direction'
'getting on with the work'
'institutional
commitment'
'brown nosing'
'blagging'
'doing your share'
'an easy life'
'respect'
'figure head'
'an aura'
'protect'
'good team player'
'duty to climb the ranks'
'sorting things out'

Status
leadership
experience
authority
'earned respect from
similar grades'
'know what you're doing'
'remaining calm'
'give advice'
'a sense of dignity'
'self-respect'
'respect from others'
'listening'
'being considerate'
'consistent interactions'
'a sense of achievement'
'a sense of role'
'status is a personal thing'
'personality type'
'confidence'
'not panicking'
'putting on a front'
'can be relied on'
'being in pro-active
alliances'
'doing the rough jobs'
'keeping stumm'

Machoness
Masculine
Hard
Non-emotional
Opposite to Feminine
Bully
Strong Body
Expected
Defensive/not thinking
Logical/lack of emotions
Loud/doing nothing
Dominant
Boisterous
Loyal/being one of the boys
'fitting in'
'not being taken seriously'
'by being a lad'
'acting the fool'
'loudly'
'male chauvinists'
'telling dirty jokes'
'by pretending to be
something you're not'
'a false front'
'being like a man'
'bouncing around—
throwing your weight
around'

Figure 9.2: Simulating difference

male and this can never be disguised. Therefore, to consume an identity becomes one of constantly needing to firm up the boundaries and stipulate the conditions by which difference is seen to be natural, an essential prerequisite, and a predetermined biological constraint that has to be actively performed.

So these must be a performance of active (re)production, an activating of difference, and of stereotypes from the wider simulated reality. Male nurses are required to moan and cringe at the male nurse portrayal in soap operas and defend, with honour, the sanctity of instincts that are biologically masculine. These are what the mythical claims of maleness are founded on.

Masculinity in terms of self-identification is thought of as being a natural phenomenon. It exists and determines how men should act, regardless of the professional boundaries. It also allows these typical behaviours and stereotypes to become actualised, but it also enforces that these are the expected norm. However, masculinity, more broadly understood, will encompass the idea that there are diverse other 'masculinities' that may be considered and taken seriously by way of self-identification. These include the idea of being caring, thoughtful and kind, because that is what nurses are.

Difference is a key principle in cultural studies. Without it no signs would have meaning. The contrast principle, which guided the development of taxonomies, serves the same purpose in the semiotic analysis of cultural knowledge. It is difference that maleness maintains with its myths of naturalness, inner cores, and universalism. Nurses tell how they respect 'difference' in the cultural sense, but the myths of gender difference will continue to provide a space for debate. The following conclusion will identify and summarise the overall impact of this discussion and research study.

Chapter 10
Summarising the themes and myths

Trained male nurses were allowed membership of the RCN for the first time in 1960.

90% of male nurses in the psychiatric case studies are members of Unison.

Musing on the Nursing discourse.

The impact of maleness

The sections in this chapter aim to summarise the themes about maleness. They all focus on 'the impact of maleness' in psychiatric nursing culture. If we remember that the semantic relationship, 'Maleness is a way to do nursing', was devised during a three-year study, then it appears that the author is speculating that maleness, as a cultural concept, has an impact or effect on nursing culture. The degree or intensity of the impact can only be surmised, but it is argued that maleness has an impact on nursing in at least two ways: (i) on the subject via subjectivization; and (ii) in affecting the ideologies (myths) of cultural knowledge.

Therefore, there are a number of central concepts that include the concepts of identity, cultural knowledge, individuality, the notion of *difference*, symbolism, and collective identity. These six concepts belong to mainstream sociology by means of their ideological nature in cultural studies. They are also important facets of maleness and related to the way an individual is positioned, via cultural knowledge, by ideological discourse. The issues of freedom and agency are the main threads running through these conceptual themes, and there is a focus on the social, cultural, and ideological impact of maleness as an effect on individual nurses who work in the same culture.

Maleness is a way to do nursing

The six ethnographic themes

- Status is a way to do maleness
- Power and hierarchy is used to do maleness
- Machoness is an attribute of maleness
- Vulnerability is a result of maleness
- Non-femaleness is used to do maleness
- Institutions are a result of maleness

Maleness [as] a way to do nursing can be identified as a theoretical position that allowed for the development of six ethnographic cultural themes. There are, of course, other possible themes, but, with regards to the domain maleness, all the folk terms collected in the study are encapsulated within the six domains noted above. The following questions about the impact of maleness on psychiatric nursing culture have guided the discussion during throughout this book.

1.	What is the impact (use) of maleness on identity?	(Status)
2.	What is the impact (use) of maleness on the self?	(Vulnerability)
3.	What is the impact (use) of maleness on individuality?	(Power)
4.	What is the impact (use) of maleness on symbolism?	(Machoness)
5.	What is the impact (use) of maleness on collective identity?	(Institutions)
6.	What is the impact (use) of maleness on difference?	(Non-femaleness)

Figure 10.1: Questioning the use of maleness

Pulling it all together

Maleness reflects all that 'masculinity in psychiatric nursing' is perceived to be by the mental health nurses from the three case studies. It is a concept, which, it can be argued, has an impact on psychiatric nursing culture. First, there is the impact on the individual/subject through a process of *subjectivization*. Second, there is sustained impact, via this subjectivization, of individuals in producing *cultural knowledge* by exchanging representations (symbols) that have meaning.

Maleness has an affect on their individual identity that can be observed in the way the male body is given peculiar status. A body that is actively reproducing and 'masquerading' the symbolism (myths) of individuality, as understood to have meaning in psychiatric culture. This subjectivization seemingly occurs without the subjects knowledge, and subjects conform in order to 'position the self' and avoid misrepresenting 'a performance of self'. Thus, the issue of power and sex type theories allow for a significant insight into how informants in psychiatric nursing culture view the representation of gender types. The relevance of power is discussed as being a force that is not subjectively owned by individuals, but rather, a network of relationships constituted by discourse acting *on* individuals, rather than by individuals.

From the analysis of the six domains of maleness, it is possible to identify at least nine myths that reoccur again and again throughout nursing culture. These myths focus on maleness and nursing culture and are now summarised:

Myth 1: Each nurse performs the way they do because they choose to. They are autonomous and free thinking. Their identity is founded on a personal inner core. *An essence;*

Myth 2: There is a *natural and truthful reality* 'out there' that has objectivity;

Myth 3: Gender traits are *biologically determined* and not able to be changed;

Myth 4: Male nurses (as caring professionals) are more in touch with their 'feminine side';

Myth 5: Power is seen to be a thing that can be given; a tool that can be exercised by individuals who have it in them to maintain authority;

Myth 6: There is a simple relationship of reflection between oneself (self-identity) and an objective, real, pre-existing, universal, truthful world;

Myth 7: Meaning and truth is unchanging due to its relationship with the constant reality 'out there' that can be objectively engaged with;

Myth 8: This constant reality is objectively true and a yardstick from which all objectivity and subjectivity can be compared and understood (universalised);

Myth 9: There are naturally occurring traits, ensuring that nursing is better suited for females, such as nurturing, caring, and being sensitive.

Status is a way to do maleness (identity)

Point 1 *Male nurse status in psychiatric nursing culture is a product of subjectivization. The domain: 'Status is a way to do maleness' demonstrates how a sense of identity is partly a result of myths about maleness.*

The issue of identity is the significant ethnographic and cultural theme for this book. It recurs again and again due to its relationship with both the focal data and the interpretative nature of the thesis development. As a starting point, the ethnographic concept of status provides a domain of maleness enabling the researcher to put forward the argument that maleness can be said to constitute a seemingly stable sense of identity for male nurses.

Point 2 *Male nurses feel free to create any identity they want, but, in practice, they are pushed (and push themselves) towards identities representing the perceived values of nursing cultural knowledge. These representations are produced and consumed, therefore, maintaining the dominant cultural meaning.*

This is evident in the following discussion. Male nurses believe they arrive at an identity, which is 'natural' and determined as a result of their individual history and personality traits. Yet, they are subjected to conform to those performances that have meaning in nursing culture, i.e., they will abide and perform the masquerades of nursing and maleness discourse.

Point 3 *Contrary to the general assumption held by the nurse informants, maleness seems to produce representations of what it is to be a male nurse. It provides dif-*

ferent identities and, therefore, a different status for male nurses.

It is the signs and symbols, and their meaning in psychiatric nursing culture, which constitute identity, not *vice versa.* It is assumed, by the informants, that they are individuals with 'unique identities' who impose themselves on the culture, yet this point allows for a different interpretation: that nursing culture has a number of sought-after symbols of status prescribed and aspired to by nurses.

Point 4   *The body, as a status object, denies the possibility of individual identity for men and, thus, supports the earlier proposition that they are trapped in their representations.*

The notion of individuality is denied by the fact that, physically, all male nurses carry the symbolism of maleness. Identity has to be constituted within these parameters. It will be argued that an alternative interpretation of individuality can be uncovered from the signs and symbols of nursing culture.

Point 5   *Male nurses are active reproducers of gender behaviours; they (re)produce and masquerade maleness as an identity and are, in themselves, not free agents. They are not outside of cultural meaning.*

The criteria for how maleness can be used is already determined by nursing culture. Male nurses are active in its reproduction of performance and the identities they masquerade. Some are moody, some are fun, some are good at care planning and, therefore, seemingly different; yet there remains a cultural expectation based upon the 'symbolism' they perform/represent.

Vulnerability is a result of maleness (the self)

Point 6   *The notion of spectatorship and subjectivization is founded on the way discourses are the bearers of various historically specific positions of agency and identity for nurses. It is these subject-positions that provide the conditions for subjects to act, or have 'knowledge' in relation to particular social practices.*

All men are not equal. Maleness and nursing discourse provides the positions for nurses to occupy. This is best related to the notion of vulnerability and power.

Point 7 *'Vulnerability is a result of maleness' is a domain, which, like others, can allow for an examination of the emergence of modern forms of individuality through the growth of new bodies of knowledge and networks of power. It is possible to see the representations of sex role traits of male nurses as marking the formation of a new subject-position for men.*

Power and hierarchy are used to do maleness (individuality)

Point 8 *Nurses can only have knowledge of things if they have cultural meaning. It is discourse—not the things in themselves—that produce knowledge. Knowledge is put to work through discursive practices to regulate the conduct of others.*

Point 9 *Power operates within institutional apparatus and its technologies, the assumption being that 'psychiatry needs men'. However, male nurses are not more powerful as subjects (than the other); they are representing maleness, which is more powerful in power's circulation.*

Point 10 *Power is productive in the constitution of maleness through specific visual codes and forms of looking. It fixes the boundaries between the normal and the abnormal (binary oppositions of maleness).*

The idea that power is a neutral entity, as opposed to 'an authority' that individuals have, hides the concept that individuals are constituted within systems of meaning that have a moral or ethical *connotation*. The moral message is usually one that says, 'this is the way we do it here'. Therefore, one set of symbols will have a privileged position within a culture above all other signs.

Point 11 *The starting point for understanding maleness lies, not in the contrast with femininity, but in the asym-*

metric dominance and prestige that belongs to male nurses in their given cultures.

Issues of power can be interpreted from the prestige that male nurses enjoy in their daily performances in nursing culture.

Point 12   *Male nurses are located in their maleness by power, which subjectifies them. This seems to make certain forms of agency and individuality appear more stable. However, subjectivization does not require individual male nurses to be interpellated through mechanisms of identification to secure the workings of power/knowledge over them.*

The following points concern cultural issues. In particular, the relationship of symbolism, as a constructing force in the policing of cultural knowledge. The use of machoness, in the clinical setting, is given as an example of how maleness maintains a certain cultural meaning related to how male nurses are expected to perform their everyday, masculine rituals. This is summarised with an exploration into the defining boundaries of where maleness ends—with the identification of 'the other'—the female. The idea that male nurses aim to be non-female helps us to understand that the impact of maleness on nursing, not only defines the identity of male individuals, but also all nurses and, on a cultural level, the entire psychiatric nursing profession.

Machoness is an attribute of maleness (symbolism)

Point 13   *All signs are arbitrary—there is no natural relationship between the sign and its meaning or concept. Signs themselves cannot fix meaning. Meaning is relational. There is no simple relationship of reflection, imitation, or one-to-one correspondence between language and the real world.*

Point 14   *Representation is the production of meaning through symbols.*

It seems that there is no better substitute than machoness (properly termed machismo (Oxford Dictionary)) for identifying the significant symbolism of 'what it is to be a male'. Symbolism—the use of signs makes use of cultural knowledge and codes.

Institutions are a result of maleness (collective identity)

Point 15   *Nursing openly promotes certain norms of behaviour, while covering up innately human issues by not acknowledging them. The representation of maleness as an identity is such an issue. Yet maleness is a simulation, it is of auto-identification, parody and masquerade of symbolic representations.*

The issue of ideology and myths of nursing culture can be realised by exploring the issues of performance, masquerades, and simulation. These concepts, taken from post-structural theory, enable an interpretation that questions the very existence of nursing 'truth'.

Non-femaleness is used to do maleness (difference)

Point 16   *Women represent a limit of the male symbolic order; a frontier to the phallogocentric nursing cultural meaning of maleness.*

Male status is not the same as female status regardless of the profession's attempt to naturalise, universalise, and essentialise cultural knowledge.

Point 17   *Masculinity does not exist in isolation from femininity—it will always be an expression of the current image men have of themselves (auto-identification) in relation to women. At any given moment, gender identities will reflect the material interests of those who have power, and those who do not.*

Ideology is seen as a set of beliefs, not necessarily made about what nurses think, but how they act and how the nursing profession expects representation to occur. Therefore, the three themes of machoness, institutions and non-femaleness all appear to be challenging and an uncomfortable thorn in the side of this representation. This is due, in part, to the fact that these themes belong to the non-opposing, yet distinct discourse of maleness.

Summary

The aim of this chapter was to summarise the discussion points presented in the previous chapters. The important points to consider are: the ideas of (i) subjectivization, (ii) cultural knowledge, and (iii) the myths of nursing and maleness that attempt to naturalise, essentialise, universalise, and underplay the importance of marginalised competing ideologies.

Chapter 11
Boys will be boys—conclusions

'Nearly all the early research and theoretical debate specifically concerned with the sociology of gender focussed on women and femininity. In recent years it has been recognised that a more complete understanding of gender can be developed by also studying men and masculinity'.

(Haralambos and Holborn, 1995, p581)

This chapter aims to conclude the themes of the book and the major points it has advanced. In order to do this it will also describe that which the study and book has **not** advanced. This chapter will conclude what implications the study might have for how nursing can advance the subject area of gender and cultural studies in the future.

Why study male nurses?

The original study aims were developed to explore what can be termed 'traditional' subject matter in gender and cultural studies. That is, they aimed to *explore the extent of congruence between male and female nurses' perceptions of nursing culture.* It was expected that the case study design would confirm the existence of sociologically-defined, gender-related traits, which could account for *differences* between male and female psychiatric nurses. However, within the first three weeks of collecting data, the author began to realise that his original aims, although feasible, were narrow and elementary. These original aims set an agenda, which assumed that biological sex difference could account for certain traits in nursing practice, one that took, as its starting point, an assumption that, in wider society, men are the norm against which women are comparable. Therefore, in a female-dominated profession, it seemed more useful to explore how male nurses adapt, create identities and demonstrate *difference* behaviourally.

By week three in Case 1, the author was beginning to realise that these specific differences in behavioural traits were not as forthcoming as the literature would suggest. It seemed that psychiatric nursing culture was, in part, responsible for the reproduction of gender relations that kept masculinity invisible. The *difference* seemed to be all around, but mostly in relation to how male nurses made sense of their own identity, an identity that exaggerated the universal and essential properties of their biological sex. The author began to believe, during these early stages, that nursing culture and gender identity, when studied ethnographically, could produce a modest range of ethnographic taxonomies that reflected gender issues for the nurses. These issues could be thought of as signs and symbols of representation. Therefore, the aim of identifying specific gender trait differences needed to be revised and new aims that focussed on the impact of these symbols in nursing culture developed.

The revised aim was *to describe the cultural conditions and the context that related to the practice of male psychiatric nurses and to identify the key ethnographic themes of gender and their relationship to issues of masculinities for male nurses.* This aim paid more attention to the cultural space in which male nurses represented their masculinity by way of signs. The study of this cultural space made it possible for the researcher to consider the use of a semiotic and post-structural analysis of cultural ideologies in which these masculine signs resided. Retrospectively, it is possible to see that the aims of the study, the theoretical issues, and the methods needed to achieve the aims had progressed with the use of the DRS. In this sense, it is plausible to conclude that the study, not only achieved its aim of describing the cultural conditions and developing ethnographic themes, but also provided a discussion that took into account post-structural theory to advance a contribution focussed on psychiatric nursing culture. The author's groundwork required him to record the thousands of included terms, taxonomies, and the significant six domains of maleness from which the ethnographic themes were interpreted.

Practical changes in data collection

To conclude that the data collection methods employed by the author at the start of the study were wholly successful would be an exaggeration. Although the use of the case study method enabled the fulfilment of the study aims, some changes to the methods of data collection were implemented. The practical application of observations and interviews required modification from the commencement of *Case 1*.

Observation

The change in the actual method centred upon the need to adapt the observation of informants into a shadowing process. As a data collection strategy, this permitted the author to be more effective and efficient with his time and use of self. He was able to develop relationships with each of the informants. The original intention was to use an observation checklist and, by doing so, attempt to standardise the data being recorded (e.g. female nurses showed more friendly non-verbal behaviours than male nurses). Also, the initial attempt at remaining in a single area to record interactions between informants proved to be more problematic than expected (e.g. interaction takes place between people as opposed to location alone). The idea of the author as a 'professional stranger' shifted the requirements of the observation away from wanting to standardise the data collected towards a more anthropological approach, which had serious consequences for the nature of the data collected. By being a 'professional stranger', the author immediately noticed the increase in data quantity and in the quality, which permitted a new way of thinking about the study. This new way of critical thinking, which was central to the development of the new aims, focussed on the possibility of exploring the signs informants made sense of, represented, and masqueraded in order to present an identity. Similarly, it enabled a more flexible and, therefore, more focussed exploration of the ways informants represented signs, which were determined within the remits of a 'hidden' nursing ideology. As the study progressed, throughout the case studies, the observations allowed the author to evolved the focus of his observation away from behavioural traits, towards specific attitudes and signs (taxonomies) and, finally, towards the existence of specific ethnographic themes about maleness.

Interviews

The collection of interview data was dependent, in part, upon the ability of the author to make use of ethnographic questioning. As he grew more confident and expert with the Developmental Research Sequence (DRS) and theoretical implications of the systemic structural theory, the nature of data changed. The analysis of data in tandem proved to be more complex and, on occasions, was not feasible. However, despite this, the analysis of data during what became known as Phase One (using taxonomies and domains) proved to be effective, even if it was costly in terms of time and the 'mundane' (Spradley, 1979). It also emphasised the use of the 'researcher as a tool', which had an impact on the author. He had, originally, not given this facet much thought, but it became clear that the interviews for the study were producing data, which was useful and yet dependent upon the methods the author was able to demonstrate in order to make the most from each interaction with informants. The author could not remained detached; he became a professional stranger who was developing his interviewing skills as the study progressed. Therefore, the interviewing process was about change and development, which impacted upon the researcher. This is an important conclusion, because the objectivity of scientific method is brought into question. The data and the interpretation of it belongs to the researcher in the objective sense, but to conclude that the interview data is subjective would be equally wrong. The process of layering and developmental evolution (sequence), which the interviews demonstrate, emphasise the idea that ethnographic interviewing is an investment. This feeling of investing in the method of ethnographic interviewing is a conclusion that was not anticipated prior to the study, but has had a powerful effect on the author's attitude to his work and his informants' working lives.

Myths

The 'translating' of myths, identified from the taxonomies, was an exciting prospect for the author. The applied semiotic and post-structural theory enabled him to interpret data from psychiatric nursing culture in a novel and original way. In particular, the significance of cultural knowledge and subjectivization reflected a more radical and challenging interpretation of how male nurses made sense of their identity. It signalled a move away from traditional attempts to stimulate more traditional gender research (about *difference*), towards a more critical appraisal of nursing culture as a whole. It also signified a progression into a scientific area that has many controversial pitfalls. The use of 'interpretation' can be viewed as being non-scientific and open to fierce debate.

The theoretical perspectives

There have been a number of theoretical foundations upon which this book has relied. This section of the conclusion will subject each one of them to a brief examination to evaluate their usefulness and impact during the study.

The importance of sex role theory and the plethora of previous research suggests that this study might have progressed in a well worn path, a path that would have attempted to emphasise *difference* in the various attributes relevant to each of the sexes within psychiatric nursing culture. This may have been useful in some respects, but it would have also served to promote a distinction between the two sexes. This type of theoretical approach has been the traditional starting point for much of the gender research.

For the outcomes of this study, the sex role theory helped to emphasise that this is an area, which is under-researched in nursing and one that has many exciting research possibilities. In particular, it enabled the researcher to pursue the idea of large ideologies in nursing culture associated with gender roles and cultural identity. The issue of cultural *identity* is central to the study (as opposed to the idea of *difference*). It allowed the author to consider the reasons why earlier gender research dictated that which could be deemed useful and, therefore, researchable.

By emphasising difference as the primary consideration, sex role theory attempts to deny the plausibility of other (namely social constructionist) perspectives, which have become more dominant in recent post-feminist gender research. The issue of biological determinism that has dominated gender research (especially in the ideas we have about 'identity') can be explored and interpreted using a different political and moral agenda.

Therefore, the sex role theory is still considered to be an important influence on how many people perceive and account for the gender expectations and biological attributes associated with men and women. Within the gender research field, this book is now part of what seems to be a growing concern for exploring cultural, ideological, and power issues. Sex role theory was useful in helping the author to discover the possibility of the powerful dynamics and ideologies, which have gone to promote this type of 'difference' research as useful and dominant. Sex role theory demands different questions and centres its aims distinctly.

This book has gone someway in examining the reliance people place on binary thinking to help ensure a sense of stable identity for themselves, and as a model to reduce the uncertainty of life experiences. Structural theory, as developed during the last one hundred years, has aimed to provide a scientific approach to understanding language and its structuring effects on social beings.

The idea of the myth gives a template (a credible and recognised template) to the study of culture. The premise is, that because all meaning is situated in language, then culture can be analysed using semiotic principles. The importance of the myth, as a theoretical anchor and framework, allowed this study to progress from the Spradley (1979) structural approach to the Barthes (1996) post-structural. This transition, it should be concluded, was made simple due to the epistemological overlap of the two. In addition, the idea of the myth enabled the exploration of other areas of post-modern interest, such as Baudrillard (1994) and Buchbinder (1998).

This application of a post-structural perspective of nursing culture appears to be limited and in its infancy.

The limits of Barthes' usefulness were recognised by the author, as being more about the difficulty of transferring his theoretical positions into meaningful and applicable knowledge. He gave a fresh and novel method for exploring cultural phenomena. He also identified the theoretical danger that comes with it. This danger is the nature of theoretical interpretation, which social scientists have to push forward against positivist parameters of scientific credibility. The identification of other post-structuralist theorists enabled this study to progress in a manner that identifies it as being radical and at the forefront of research into gender issues within psychiatric nursing culture.

Buchbinder (1998) applies Barthes' myth to the wider cultural meanings associated with masculinities. In particular, the thesis uses his idea of performance anxiety, the homophobic determinants of masculinity, and the recognition of signs in the important development of self-identity. This helped to emphasise the idea of *identity* in this study, as being the important consideration. This study provides a new way of looking at psychiatric nursing culture, a way that is not just about the typical behaviours and roles of nurses. It is about the signs and symbols, about the forces acting upon subjects, and the consumption of various identities that male nurse's masquerade in an attempt to represent their masculine identities.

Likewise, post-feminist work provides a platform and theoretical foundation from which to assert a different way of interpreting gender issues. Post-feminist theory has provided little in the way of practical research tools, but it is abundant in theoretical abstraction. In particular, it emphasises the notions of power and discourse (Foucault, 1980) and binary oppositions. The limitations of post-feminist theory for this study are that such thought is often perceived to be radical and, possibly, too psychoanalytical. Yet, it has to be acknowledged by way of conclusion, that post-feminist theorists are continuing to make significant contributions to our understanding of cultural issues, which can be seen as a direct consequence and a reply and response to sex role theory. Similarly, this study evolved as a reaction against the dominant insistence of studying gender in a functional and pragmatic way.

The overall study has contributed interpretative knowledge to an under-researched area in nursing and has given a framework and foundation for future research. It has raised the profile of gender issues in nursing by presenting two particular considerations. First, by way of the pre-existing status of gender research in nursing, its perceived usefulness, and seemingly unimportant issues when compared to other direct patient-centred research, this study, due to this limited interest in the topic area, is original. In combination with the distinct methodological originality, the study demonstrates that gender has to be considered an important phenomena, within the confines of psychiatric nursing culture, beyond the traditional sex type research. This revelation leads to the second point, which concerns the nature of signs, symbols, semiotics, and post-structuralism.

The cultural codes of gender come into play. They constitute gender identities; they constitute identity. They shape the very logic of the culture and make an impression at the site of myth. The traditional way of viewing gender issues would have a very different conclusion, perhaps that male nurses are more dominant, that they use particular behaviours and, that when compared to their female colleagues, show similar 'feminine characteristics'. This usual type of conclusion is obviously not the outcome of this study, which uses new research about cultural phenomena in psychiatric nursing culture. Instead, this study (apart from putting forward the notion of ideological myths, which constitute a subjectivization of the subject), also points up the originality of exploring gender from this culturally-based position. The examination of culture (as opposed to individual trait characteristics) reflects increasing post-structural and post-feminist influence. Therefore, the synthesis of theoretical analysis upon original data, which shares a compatible epistemology, demonstrates and enabled an original interpretation of psychiatric nursing culture.

It will be seen that the interpretation and critical analysis of the discussion could be considered limited in its analytical application; that is, a deeper analysis of a limited number of themes may have provided a deeper and clearer argument that myths exist, constitute knowledge, and dictate the subjective positions of nurses. However, it is the nature and direction of the analysis that can be claimed as original. The application of this type of approach to understanding nursing culture is a direct contradiction of the typical research questions of the past, which usually attempt to predict the attitudes, motivation and account for the behaviour of the minority of men in nursing. Then, hypotheses were being drawn from a world view, which insists that the starting point should be the individual. This study concludes that these types of gender-perceived attributes (behaviours associated to each sex) cannot be, and should not be, considered separately from the wider cultural discourses and myths that are operating within the various levels of nursing knowledge, which constitute these behaviours. This study has attempted to find a way to link the signs and symbols of, for example, motivated behaviour, as given by the informants, and show how they can be interpreted from a wider perspective as opposed to the traditional gender trait viewpoint. To this end, once again the researcher acknowledges that a critic might argue that it would have been more useful to focus on one single attribute, such as comradeship, and thoroughly analyse its implications. In his defence, the researcher refers back to the aims of the study and the explorative/interpretative nature of these aims.

Psychiatric nursing culture

By using a structural and post-structural methodology, it has been possible to make a particular type of analysis of a particular type of data. The degree to which this interpretation and data taken from the case study sites is useful has to be seen against the backdrop of other comparable research studies. The traditional perspectives may consider function, experience, and motive as key theoretical concepts to understanding the nature of psychiatric culture. This study has not done that in the strictest sense. Theoretically, it has offered an alternative perspective to the nature of male nurse identity/

consumption and production of nursing identity. It has 'examined myths', searched and located hundreds of gender related symbols, and interpreted the connotations of these in psychiatric nursing culture. Therefore, the originality of the study derives from the conviction that psychiatric nursing culture can be studied and explored, as a collection of cultural relationships, powerful dynamics, and collective identities. The uncertain persona of this conclusion points up the possibility that this study challenges the traditional models and beliefs regarding what nursing culture is, how it functions and the space it creates for subjects.

The issue of representation, the production and consumption of signs is a particular area for consideration. The originality consists in the application of these at a conceptual, as well as a methodological level. To interpret psychiatric nursing culture in terms of signs/symbols and production/consumption is an outcome of this thesis. The conclusion, therefore, emphasises that this study should be viewed as the start of continuing research, because it cannot be conclusive at this theoretical level. The ethnographic themes and taxonomies from Phase One provide a firmer base from which psychiatric nursing culture can be seen as a closed system, which consumes a certain number of symbols that pertain to a certain type of enclosed knowledge. The meaning of signs and symbols are seen to be universalised, essential and based upon humanistic theoretical foundations. This can be concluded with more certainty, yet the idea that these foundations are made up of ideological myths in which signs are consumed cannot be so conclusive.

What the study has helped support

The principle theory that the study has applied and supported is both structuralist and post-structuralist theory from a number of theorists. These include ideas about cultural studies and gender, and approaches to understanding them advocated by Barthes, Buchbinder, Foucault, Sassure, Strauss, Hall, post-feminist writers, such as Kristeva, Kitzinger and Irigaray, psychoanalytical concerns about masculinity, Tolson, and the work of Mac an Ghaill and Connell. It should be concluded that these theorists share a common concern in the paradigm of social constructionism and do not necessarily agree. Yet, they are important theorists who are pioneers in the application of structural and post-structural theory. Thus, this study has relied upon their contributions to progress.

In particular, the use of the DRS has helped to support the use of semiotics in practice. By doing so, it has enabled the use of consistent terms, particularly those of Foucault, Barthes and Buchbinder. The application of semiotics and post-structural analysis, within this topic area, has supported the view that identity should be viewed as a fragmented theoretical concern.

The study has also opened up the possibility of applying radical ideas regarding consumption, identity, and masquerade to a culture that has little insight into these issues. It should be concluded, therefore, that the use of structural and post-structural theories has been fully implemented at both a methodological and theoretical level during the study. This opens up the possibility of further use in the future. This alternative approach gives more breadth to an area of nursing, mostly consider either poorly researched, or an insignificant priority.

By raising an awareness of larger structures (ideologies), which impact upon nursing culture and informants, this work is consistent with other attempts to destabilise universal grand narratives and, therefore, contradict many of the emic and theoretical assumptions informants hold about the nature of their gender identity, their cultural knowledge, and their sense of a truthful reality. This is a contentious area of debate and one that this study has not sought to resolve. Instead, it has not avoided the difficult and uncomfortable associations of such post-modern theorising and has sought, instead, to raise issues and its possible analytical status through future post-structural application.

The study has given evidence to suggest that the study of psychiatric nursing culture can successfully be researched taking into account three distinct structuralist themes. First, that all culture uses language of signs to organise and construct reality. It enables nurses to give meaning to their culture. Second, this meaning only occurs in relation to structures. Every sign is given meaning. It is not a naturally occurring event and it only has meaning in relation to other signs (contrast principle). Third, verbal and non-verbal language provides a clear demonstration of these structural or relational properties of meaning, as shown in the taxonomies of Phase One. The interpretations of Phase Two demonstrates how meaning in psychiatric nursing culture is a product of difference between signs and their consumption. This thesis has brought to the forefront difference between signs, in order to disrupt any notion of stability or unity of meaning, as opposed to the foundational (sex type) theory that attempts to account for difference as being biologically determined and, therefore, universal.

It is easy to describe the theory that this study challenges and contradicts. Those theories, which allude to discursive narratives and advocate metaphysical associations with inner essences, universalism, autonomy, and foundationalism, by their very nature are seen to be philosophical positions that are contradicted by the structural and post-structural aspirations of sociological thought. This study can be seen as bringing to the fore a number of questions about meaning, representation, and authorship, and as exploring the relationship between language and knowledge that challenges the dominant moral and value judgements associated with these philosophies. The work of the post-feminist, Kristeva (1982), highlights the central issue of this thesis regarding identity and forms of knowing, when she argues that the male-dominated society discourages multiple forms of selfhood. She holds this, partly, because our identities are confined to rigid gender definitions, which the researcher would argue has been the mainstay of most gender research to date. This biological deterministic paradigm of gender studies has been challenged by the study in the course of giving an alternative interpretation: a social constructionist interpretation as to how male nurses are subjectivised by maleness, represent maleness, and (re)produce maleness in the form of signs and symbols for consumption. This position examines the fragmented nature of identity, the determinist nature of discourse and language, and the possibility that the existence of any 'inner essence' is a subversive ideology constituted by psychiatric nursing culture.

Similarly, the issue of humanist autonomy and the grand narratives pertaining to the existence of an individual identity is challenged by the researcher's interpretation, drawn from the focal data. The idea that male nurses are able to perceive themselves as having autonomy and the ability to achieve self actualisation is interpreted by the researcher as being a myth that, itself, creates a particular type of subjectivization. The conclusions drawn from this study show that these typical notions held by male nurses are worthy of further exploration, perhaps a focus on more specific concepts, and definitely a deeper analysis before any rigours and influential conclusions could be drawn. But, having acknowledged that, this study should be considered as an initial introduction to an alternative way of understanding what psychiatric nursing culture means to male nurses.

The limitations

This book does not offer a final theory regarding the place of gender issues in psychiatric nursing culture. It does not claim to have the answers to why male nurses do what they do, or provide a model to predict their future behaviours. In some ways, these can be regarded as failures of the study, but they are better seen as limitations. By identifying these limitations, it is hoped that this conclusion can be said to be more 'conclusive' and perhaps lead the way to furthering that to which the thesis has contributed.

The topic of gender and cultural studies is large and there is no consensus of opinion. This seemingly confused starting point for the study has not been made any clearer by its outcomes. This book does not remedy any of the continuing debates between the sex type and social constructionist camps of academic theory. It never intended to, but it has, in fact, added an alternative approach to an already confused arena. The debates will continue. What this book does, is offer one interpretation regarding the identity of male nurses in psychiatric nursing culture and is, therefore, an initial attempt at defining a starting point.

The variables (concepts), or distinct lack of them due to the nature of the epistemology and methodology, makes the study appear messy and, for some, non-scientific. This is disputed, but, nevertheless, is a limitation that will make some reserve judgement regarding the usefulness of the study's findings.

Similarly, the confusion over defining some of the important concepts, such as masculinity, maleness, simulation, masquerades, reproduction, and the like, stems from the way the concepts have no generally agreed or fixed positions within cultural studies. They seem to have an opaque meaning, but this study has needed to create definitions, and these could create even more uncertainty and a reluctance by others to see the study as useful. This attempt to create definitions has limited analysis, and future research would perhaps be required to remedy this.

Therefore, the many interpretations put forward may be viewed as statements about ill-defined concepts, views about abstract and non-tangible issues, which cannot be tested scientifically. This is acknowledged, and emphasises the conceptual nature of the study.

The importance of the focal data and its relevance may be a limitation that over-stresses the properties of the data, as 'meaning' something more than they do. As such, this type of interpretation will be viewed as abstracting or stretching the meaning of the non-translated emic taxonomies too much and, therefore, denying the sophistication of statistical and other operational analysis. This is a recognised criticism, but one inherent in the study aims and the theory generating paradigm of scientific research to which this study firmly belongs.

Researcher bias is an issue; as the study progressed the author had been drawn into the paradigm of post-structural theory. Therefore, such bias has to be considered because the researcher may have overloaded and overlooked subtle concepts, significant research, or other important theory, such as symbolic interactionism, which would have created differing interpretations. It is felt that this is a plausible argument, but the focal data of this study goes more to support the theoretical issues of post-structural theory. The study was data-led not theory-led in this respect. And it occurred to the author that the aims of the study focus on cultural issues rather than on the individual, as a dynamic performer who has researchable commodities. Bearing this in mind, it has to be concluded that the theoretical persuasion of the focal data may be improved or contradicted by a future application of a more hermeneutical or grounded theory type analysis.

Generalisability (transferability) may be considered a shortcoming in regard to the taxonomic findings and the interpretations forming the discussion. The generalisability and representativeness of the findings can be seen to reflect the expected outcomes of the study. The methodology and sampling procedures were such that a predictive or, at most, correlational generalisability would be limited. However, it is recognised that this study can only be applied superficially to other settings in the strictest objective sense. It was always envisaged that future work would be able to complement and advance the findings of this work.

Where further work/analysis is needed

Even though this book feels complete up to this point, it should not mean that these conclusions are the end. A plausible new phase would have the aim of subjecting the weaker areas of this work to further analysis and research. There are a number of issues that could be expanded by this exploration.

Further analysis would be required of some interpretative points, in particular, a twofold attempt at describing the broader aspects (perhaps at a policy level) regarding the nature of maleness for the profession of nursing, and a more defined level of the subject. In order to understand the present implications of gender identities in psychiatric nursing culture, it is permissible to analyse the overall constituents of society and/or the seemingly insignificant details of how male nurses go about within their nursing cultures. This two tier approach reflects the overall path of this study in that

Phase One concerned the mundane and everyday expressions and utterances of the informants, and Phase Two concerned the large, seemingly less obvious, patterns of gender identity. A more focussed analysis on a limited number of concepts may help clarify that gender identities for male nurses are not so universal or reflective of a unified spirit of this age, but rather, a complex mass of interweaving and contradictory desires, concerns, and values.

To conclude that further analysis is needed may be considered a failure on the part of the researcher, yet, the researcher acknowledges the limitations of his broad interpretations based on the finding of his study and his unsatisfied needs to progress his work further. Future work is needed in the area of gender and cultural studies in nursing culture *per se*, but in particular the research, which would have the most impact, would more than likely be disguised as that which has a direct impact upon practice.

The future

This final part of the conclusion is the recommendation for future research. There are a number of developments that could be taken forward from the results and conclusions of this study. The application of the same study in a general nursing culture for comparison would need to be a plausible and practical proposal. Yet this seemingly simple cross pollination of methodology would bring with it certain assumptions and feasibility difficulties of its own. These may include the low number of male nurses, a questioning of the usefulness of such a study, and the need to substantiate why such a comparison would progress understanding of nursing cultural studies. Similarly, the use of additional psychiatric nursing case studies to search for a deeper understanding of the surface themes presented in this thesis would be a plausible future research proposal.

The real possibility of future research would need to focus on the issue of identity and ask research questions, such as, who needs identity? What is the nature of male subjectivity in a female dominated (sign valued) profession? It would bring into question issues of recruitment, overall strategy planning for health care provision, and the educational needs of the future nursing student population. In addition, the question, Why does the issue of identity (in particular male identity) appear to be so neglected in nursing cultural studies? All these questions are linked to what Hall and du Gay (1996) would call the critique of the self-sustaining subject at the centre of 'post-Cartesian western metaphysics'. This research, and future work related to it, seems to find itself on the edge of something new for nursing and cultural studies, generally; a paradigm of inquiry into the nature of identity in nursing as an important consideration in itself.

Future research would not only need to continue the deconstructive critique to which many of the essentialist concepts in this study have been subjected, but also refrain from attempting to supplant inadequate concepts with 'truer' ones (Hall and du Gay, 1996). It seems that future research should continue to focus on the discursive nature of ideology, related to the experience of identity, rather than 'slipping back' in attempting to focus solely on the subject. A more detailed understanding, at a theoretical level, of what 'identity' encompasses remains the aim. The semiotic approach can help forward this aim. The connotations of nurse interactions could help our thinking about identity and the production of subjectivities for working practitioners. At a practical level, this could be transferable in a research (data collection) sense to the educational setting and ritualistic procedures of nursing *per se*. In summary, future research that could be usefully guided by this work would need to ask the right questions and, just as important, ask them for the right reasons.

Chapter 12
How to explore gender issues in psychiatric nursing culture

This chapter gives an overview of the methodology and outlines the methods used during the study. It introduces the scientific application of the Developmental Research Sequence (DRS) (Spradley, 1979) and the structural analysis of data. It is intended to give the reader a brief prelude into the way the author developed his overall methodology and provide an introduction into 'how gender issues can be explored in nursing culture'.

An introduction to ethnography

As noted by Brouse (1995), 'the importance of a theoretical framework for any research study has long been recognised in the nursing literature'. The work of Fawcett (1994) highlights that only when theory directs research and research shapes theory development is science advanced. In order to be meaningful, the systematic inquiry of this study had to be guided by a conceptual framework that influenced all phases of the research process, from problem selection to data analysis. The *ethnographic* case study design provided this framework.

A search through the literature on ethnography will reveal that it is not just one approach, but what seems like hundreds of affiliated qualitative approaches. The reason for this is due, in part, to the long anthropological tradition from which ethnography, as a distinct branch, has developed. Silverman (1993) notes that Marshall and Rossman (1989) list six different qualitative research traditions, including ethnography, cognitive anthropology, and symbolic interactionism (the remaining three are not given, but would possibly include phenomenology, hermeneutics and grounded theory). These all share a commitment to naturally occurring phenomena within context, the value of peoples perceptions and experiences, and the existence of multiple realities. The theoretical and philosophical foundation of these qualitative research approaches have been the central concern of some well-known and respected academic researchers. The work of Denzin (1997) is worthy of particular note at this early stage. His analysis of ethnography has led him to, what he terms, the 'sixth moment', a moment that emphasises the post-structuralist concern for questioning 'truth' and 'reality'.

The evolutionary nature of ethnography, as a credible scientific approach, can be seen in the following research issues, which include the issues of Saussurian linguistic research (Hawkes, 1977), ethnographic induction (Bloor, 1978), observation and interviewing during field work, providing valid generalisations (Dingwall, 1980), searching for common organisational features using ethnography (Gubrium and Buckholdt, 1982), the use of transcripts in ethnographic research (Heritage 1984), collective representations of organisations (Gubrium and Holstein, 1987), the nature of articulative ethnography (Gubrium, 1988), theoretical modelling of 'seeing through the eyes of the subject' and reliability, the theoretical difficulties of artificial and natural settings (Hammersley,1992), ethnographic themes of conceptual masculinity (Gilmore, 1990), detail to ethnographic rigourousness (Sacks, 1992), and ethnographic reliability (Hammersley, 1992). These are all common issues associated with the qualitative research methodology of ethnography.

Ethnography started to be considered as a viable research methodology in nursing, due (in part) to the rise in interest of functional process models during the 1960s and 1970s. These type of models, like the 'nursing process', aim to categorise segments of experience into developing theories. Examples in nursing relate to interaction models (Peplau, 1988; Parse, 1981; Rogers, 1970), self-care models (Orem, 1991), and the individual (Parse, 1992). These few typify many others, which were emerging during this period, as an attempt to legitimise nursing through a process of scientification. The use of ethnographic and phenomenological research approaches in nursing made use of a person-centred paradigm that of humanism.

The rise of humanism has promoted a sense that sociological paradigms of science could be utilised within health care settings to provide science-based research, which could benefit direct patient care. This qualitative paradigm, with its related issues just listed, made it feasible for practitioners to implement small scale research projects emulating the work of Goffman (1961), Mead (1962), and Laing and Esterson (1964), with their shift in emphasis on the interactional and interpersonal nature of data collection and analysis. The definition of ethnography is the search for *informant emic meaning and structures of meaning* (Hammersley, 1992; Denzin, 1997) about a given culture regardless of method and data collection. However, for some, the anthropological or 'out in the field' approach is enough for the study to qualify as ethnographic. For others, there is a high degree of insight into the use of taxonomic formation and domain analysis (Spradley, 1979). As time has passed, the use of anthropological techniques, such as 'going native', devising functional categories, and the listening to life narratives, has ensured that new generations of nurses wanting to do research have been able to devise useful qualitative research projects, which are feasible in relation to their busy work loads. It is necessary to bear in mind that the literature on classic ethnography (those with older dates and non-nursing) have slowly been replaced by a type of hybrid ethnopheno-methodology that has evolved to suit the feasibility of busy nurses.

Denzin's (1997) work on interpretative ethnography can be considered one of the most important. In principle, he argues that, at this 'moment', ethnography has passed through five periods of development, which has brought us to this 'sixth moment' of ethnography. He argues that ethnography needs to be reflexive to the needs of the ethnographer and research questions. He requests that ethnographers' be creative, take risks and approach the methodology, as being distinct from positivism.

The work of Parfitt (1996), Townsend (1996), and Holland (1993) provide the most recent published works regarding the use of ethnography in nursing culture. What is striking is that, when compared to the vast numbers of phenomenological references, this is considerably smaller. However, each of the studies were conducted using Spradley's (1979) Developmental Research Sequence (DRS) as the principle framework. Therefore, they provide useful studies. All the studies highlight the historical, cultural, descriptive, and emic perspective of ethnography. Each, in turn, acknowledge the limitations of their individual studies (reliability and validity of data collection) and refer to the long standing traditions from which Spradley developed the DRS.

Reference is made by Holland to the classic contribution of Malinowski (1954) and the need to 'grasp the native's point of view', and to the work of older ethnographic studies (Aamodt, 1982; Ragucci, 1972; Byerly, 1969). Holland also acknowledges the impurity of this formulation and seems to return to Spradley's (1980) insistence of interviews and observation, seeking the mundane as an important issue of data analysis.

Parfitt (1996) used Spradley (1979) to obtain knowledge about the rules of behaviour and perceptions of informants to classify taxonomies of personal belief systems. Like Holland, she acknowledges the 'major drawbacks' of ethnoscience as perceived by positivist scientists, as not being rigorous (Field and Morse, 1991), but she cites Basso (1972), Spradley (1970), and Kay (1979) as theoretical figures in the defence of her work's rigorousness. In particular, the ethnographic model of Goodenough (1957) who, even at this early date, emphasised that cognitive processes are universal and that common structures can be identified among all cultures.

It is with the identification of 'structures' that Parfitt excels. She, unlike many, acknowledges the important contribution of Levi Strauss (1966) and Saussure (1959). She makes reference to the importance of semiological analysis (Cameron, 1985), componential analysis (Werner and Schoepfle, 1980), participant observation (Brink, 1976), and ethnographic interpretation (Nash and McCurdy, 1989), and links this to the structural development in ethnographic research.

Townsend (1996) notes how ethnography, as a research methodology, has been used to study immigration (Ng, 1984), school based education (Manicom, 1988), care provision (Campbell, 1984; Gregor, 1994), public service management (Cassin, 1990), social work (de Montigny, 1995), institutional ethnography (Douglas, 1970; Garfinkel, 1967), and the development of grounded theory (Glaser, 1978; Glasser and Strauss, 1967; Strauss and Corbin, 1990). She is not alone in her acclaim of the methodology to be considered as a serious methodology that can be adopted by university professors for their departments. For example, a quick glance through the Internet reveals university departments advertising their specialist ethnographic studies. The same is true for electronic journals (ezines) related specifically to men and masculinities.

Early publications of significant importance related to ethnography, include Freilich (1970), the previously mentioned Garfinkel (1967), which is considered one of the most substantial pieces of theory, although it is now over thirty years old. For ethnographic field work the early ethnographies provided by Kimball and Watson (1972), Spindler (1970), and of pioneering ethnographic definitions (Kroeber and Kluckhohn, 1952), and everyday ethnography's of bus riders and long distance runners (Nash, 1976; 1977), of matchbox cars (Hansen, 1976), youth sub-culture (Hewitt, 1997), American semiotics (Pierce, 1931), semantic relationships (Evans et al, 1977), distinctions in contrast questions (Conklin, 1962), ethnographic values (Spradley and McCurdy, 1975), and the concept of the ethnographic theme (Agar, 1976; 1986). A brief consideration of additional methodological issues for this study would point to the work of Lincoln and Guba (1989), particularly in relation to their insistence for establishing rigour in the qualitative research decision trail (Koch, 1994). In summary, therefore, it is possible to see that ethnography, as a qualitative methodology employing naturalistic methods of data collection, yet distinct principles of analysis, has a long and thoroughly debated history, remembering that ethnography is now in its sixth moment (Denzin, 1997).

The Developmental Research Sequence (DRS)

The DRS developed by Spradley (1979) (see *Figure 12.1* for an outline) combines well with the case study design. As noted by Merriam (1988), the case study is best suited for 'an in-depth understanding of the situation and its meaning for those involved', hence, the compatibility with the DRS. This primary consideration, of whether the philosophical and methodological assumptions of the study are congruent, meant identifying a philosophical foundation (structuralism), methodology (ethnography), and methods (case study), which were internally consistent. This relates to five major philosophical paradigmatic assumptions and considerations. (1) A belief in multiple realities; (2) The importance of the con text of a phenomenon; (3) A non-causal model; (4) The experiences of people; and (5) Analysis based on words rather than numbers. In addition, as noted by Dickson (1995), the assumptions of the method selected should be consistent with the research question: in this case, the exploring of masculinities in nursing culture.

The DRS allows for the basic assumption that people assign meaning to their world via contact with cultural knowledge. For the ethnographer, this enables a concern for local meaning to generate knowledge about specific culture, the aim being to discover meaning and understanding, rather than verify truth or predict outcomes. It is 'research with people, rather than on people' (Dickson, 1995). Lincoln and Guba (1985) have described this as, 'naturalistic inquiry', a common term, which requires certain principles to be adhered to in order to be scientifically credible. Therefore, before considering the principle analytical stages of the DRS (methods of data collection, domain analysis, taxonomic analysis, and componential analysis), the following section considers the methodological issues: (i) Sampling, and (ii) Credibility and Trustworthiness.

Sampling: (Stage 1) Locating the informant and (Stage 2) Engaging the informant

This section describes the underlying sampling principles adopted during data collection.

There are two basic approaches to sampling: (1) probability; and (2) non-probability sampling (Talbot, 1995). The randomness of probability sampling offers the advantages of being the most representative, therefore, allowing more accurate generalisation to the target population. Non-probability sampling has the advantage of being less expensive and more time-efficient. Both these approaches belong to the positivist paradigm of scientific discovery and, although capable of maximising generalisabilitity and representativeness, are not a prerequisite in ethnographic inquiry. At its closest, the study made use of non-probability sampling because of its feasibility. There are three types of non-probability sampling: (1) convenience sampling; (2) quota sampling; and (3) purposive sampling. The study made use of the latter, which, according to Glasser and Strauss (1967), is sometimes called 'judgmental' or 'theoretical sampling'. As noted by Talbot (1995), the researcher, based on knowledge and expertise of the subject, selects or 'hand-picks' the elements of the study. The elements chosen are thought to best represent the phenomenon or topic being studied. The decision to use a non-random sample (purposeful sampling) for the study required that a number of specific sampling procedures were adhered to. These will now be discussed in relation to the case study methodology.

Population

A population refers to a group whose members possess specific attributes. Therefore, the population may consist of events, places, objects, animals, or individuals (Talbot, 1995). In research, two populations are described: (1) the target population; and (2) the accessible population. The target population for this study was nurses practising within psychiatric institutional settings or ward cultures. The accessible population was the target population group to which the author had access. These nurses, known as informants, were those who

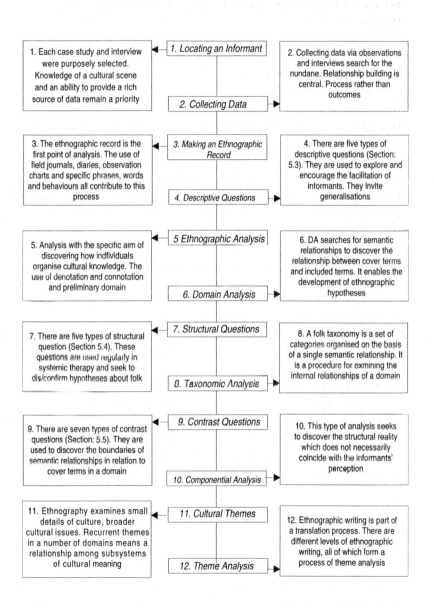

Figure 12.1: The Developmental Research Sequence (DRS) (Stages from Spradley, 1979; Descriptions adapted by the authorStages used in the study

participated in the three case studies and the male nurses who were willing to part take in additional interviews.

The issue of parameter, random sampling, and representativeness in the sampling process was considered in terms of the underlying structural methodology. For the purpose of the study, random selection as a process of selecting a representative sample of the target population was not a high priority. Nevertheless, the case study sites and the individual nurses who participated in the interviewing were mostly unknown to the author prior to the study and were chosen for their perceived ability to provide data. Each was selected after the previous case study had been completed. The issue of representativeness, that is, how well the sample represents the variables of interest in the target population was considered to be attained by collecting in-depth data reflecting, what Patton (1990) notes as, one of the greatest differences between qualitative and quantitative approaches, i.e., the different logics that underlie sampling methods. 'Qualitative inquiry typically focuses in-depth on relatively small samples, even in single cases ($n = 1$)'. The technique of using purposefully selected informants suited the aims of the study, which can be seen as typical of ethnographic methodological design (Hammersley, 1992).

The sampling process of the study necessitated an emphasis on both what to sample and how to sample. The study followed the work of Kuzel (1992) and Spradley (1979), in that the DRS, as its title suggests, is a developmental sequence, a sequence that has the following characteristics:

1. The sample design, although preconceived (at least enough to answer the question, Where and with whom do I start?), is flexible and evolves as the study progresses;

2. Sample 'units' are selected serially. Who and what comes next depends on who and what came before;

3. The sample is adjusted continuously by the concurrent development of theory. (The decision to facilitate in-depth interviews, as opposed to a fourth case study, reflects this consideration);

4. Selection continues to a point of redundancy;

5. Sampling includes a search for negative causes (disconfirming evidence), in order to give developing theory greater breadth and strength. (This was made feasible using ethnographic hypothesis and the nature of ethnographic questioning—where all sampled data is seen to be useful).

Reliability & Validity = Credibility & Authenticity: (Stage 3) Principles of the ethnographic record

Reliability or *credibility* of ethnographic data is ensured in a number of ways. In particular, the first principle is the establishment of good rapport with informants, which ensures that they are more likely to co-operate and be truthful. A second method made use of checking what the group thinks, by asking the informants, first, what they think and then, what they believe the group thinks (structural questions); also, repeat the questions with different informants to see if you have it right (testing *ethnographic hypotheses*). The use of repeated observations and interviews, by the author, enabled credible data to be collected, data that was authentic to other male nurses, and easily recognised as being truthful to their 'reality'. This, according to Goetz and Lecompte (1984), reminds researchers that 'Validity is [in ethnography] concerned with accuracy of scientific findings'. It requires: (1) Determining the extent to which conclusions effectively represent empirical *reality*; and (2) confirming whether constructs devised by researchers represent or measure the categories of human experience that occur. Therefore, to fully participate in the DRS, Spradley (1979) suggests that informants should fulfil a number of criteria so that an *ethnographic record* can be established. These criteria attempt to provide credibility to the methods employed to collect data, and also ensure that the ethnographic themes drawn are authentic. This study ensured this by maintaining that the sample of nurses were; (i) familiar with their nursing culture (e.g. not just started or agency nurses); (ii) were fully involved in that setting; (iii) could give time for the interviews; (iv) were representative of the community group. All the nurses, who participated in the case studies, fulfilled these criteria.

The ongoing stages of the Developmental Research Sequence.

Denzin (1997), Tuck (1995), Spradley (1979; 1980), Werner and Schoepfle (1987), and Agar (1986) are just some of the most popular advocates of ethnographic research. They have described, in detail, the complex process of ethnography, including the sampling, credibility, and representations of results. An important part of the ethnographic process, which is constantly emphasised, is the belief that analysis should occur simultaneously with data collection. The two are seen as an on-going process, dependent on each other to ensure meaning from a culture can be extracted using preceding data. The collection of data (using *descriptive, structural,* and *contrast questions*) necessitates analysis that, in turn, creates more avenues for increasingly focussed data collection. Hence, the preceding sampling model, advocated by Kuzel (1992). The data collected from *Case 1* was that related to the broad question: 'What behavioural gender differences can be observed in practice?' and, 'What gender differences do nurses of both sexes feel are apparent in this culture?' The answers allowed the researcher to analyse and formulate other broad questions for *Case 2*: 'Are the observable gender differences comparable to those of *Case 1*?' and, 'Why do all the informants seem to share common assumptions regarding behavioural traits, common stereotypes, and cultural expectations?'

The analysis of data from *Case 1* informed the collection and subsequent analysis of *Case 2*, which, in turn, provided questions, such as: 'What effect do masculinity(ies) have on the way male nurses perform their everyday nursing duties?', 'How do male nurses re-produce expected masculine traits?' and, 'What meaning does legitimising masculine traits have for male nurses?' Thus, the development of more focussed and abstract questions informed the researcher as to what type of structural questions the informants should be asked. The huge amount of data necessitated a growing and complex management system of in and out trays, and computer software. However, as noted 25 years ago by Bogdan and Taylor (1975), 'it is during the post-field stage of the research that [the researcher] concentrates most on the analysis and interpretation of data'. In between *Case 1* and until the termination of *Case 2*, the author had spent a total of eight months constantly sifting through notes, becoming totally immersed in the data.

This continual analysis and data management started identifying themes. Using ethnographic hypotheses, the researcher was able to search for more focussed data regarding a particular issue. For example, the way female nurses always sat down on seats during handovers compared to male nurses, who would sit on the floor or occupy higher positions, perched upon desks, swinging their legs. Was this observation to do with the representation of masculinity, as the interview themes would suggest, or was it simply to do with the wearing of skirts? The analysis, which took place after the collection of data and the termination of the three case studies, sought to provide firmer themes and interpretations.

An overview : Descriptive, structural and contrast questions

Wilson (1985), as noted by Mariano (1995), argues that there are two major purposes of data analysis in qualitative research. The questions generated for each case study reflect these purposes. The first is to *explore and describe*, the second, to *discover and explain*. These two transpired as the researcher actively searched the data to discover core patterns, transferences, and concepts that become the basis for generating hypothetical statements related to maleness. The DRS process of analysis follows 12 distinct stages as identified in *Figure 12.1*. The use of descriptive questions is given as stage 5 in the DRS, yet descriptive questions, as with all ethnographic questions, are used by the ethnographer when appropriate. The early use of descriptive questions is to elicit descriptive data from informants, from which general included terms and themes can be located.

The task of structural questions alongside descriptive questions is to confirm the use of folk terms. Questions, such as, What are all of the ways male nurses 'play the fool'? and What are all of the results of 'being in charge'? are examples of structural questions that are asked of all informants. The answers to these type of questions, in turn generate new questions, such as: 'What are all the results of bossing nurses around' and 'What are the attributes of 'being a joker'? As one might expect, there is a considerable amount of overlap between the answers of these questions, but it is this complex web of semantics that can be engaged using contrast questions to distinguish differences between included terms and their subsets.

An overview of the analytic process

There are numerous approaches to analysing qualitative data (of which at least 26 are noted by Tesch (1990)) and all have different analytical focus. Mariano (1995) states that these approaches include content/textual analysis, analytic induction, hermeneutic analysis, aesthetics, matrix analysis, constant comparison, phenomenological analysis, quasi-judicial analysis, ethnographic, and reflection. All these can be divided into two distinct groups. First, structural analysis and secondly, interpretational analysis. The analysis of the case studies took the form of structural analysis of language and behaviour (symbols and signs) to discover meaning and semantic relationships between signs.

Stages 6 (Domain Analysis), 8 (Taxonomic Analysis) and 10 (Componential Analysis) are founded on structural epistemology. These three types of analysis rely on the premise that cultural knowledge is created by the use of symbols; a symbol being an object, behaviour, or event that refers to something else. For example, 'machoness' is a symbol. All symbols have three elements: (i) the symbol; (ii) one or more referents; and (iii) a relationship between the symbol and the referent. The symbols are named by the informants and called *folk terms*. The symbol 'machoness' may have a universal meaning or referential meaning, defining it as someone who is a man, undeniably heterosexual, and possibly aggressive. However, the symbol also has referred meanings, such as: someone who is non-feminine, not in touch with their emotions, stereotypically predictable, not caring, and alien to mental health nursing. It also includes connotations (the second level and post-structural analysis of myth) of old fashioned psychiatric nursing, a lack of professionalism, and poor awareness and personal insight. As can be seen, there are many plausible referents for every symbol.

The referent alone cannot decode the meaning of the symbol. It is necessary to identify the relationship between the referent and the symbols. As noted by Parfitt (1996), these relationships are semantic. Referents are related to each other because they are linked with the symbol. Once linked with a symbol, they are called categories. A category is a group of distinct things that are equivalent, i.e., they are all equally related to a symbol, although they may be related in different ways through the semantic relationship. Referents also act as symbols with referents of their own.

Domain analysis (Stage 6)

A domain is the overall term given to a symbolic category. The first component within a domain is the cover term. Cover terms are names for a category of knowledge; for example, 'maleness' is the cover term for this book and, like all domains, it has a second component: the included term. All domains have one or more included terms, which belong to the category of knowledge named by the cover term. For example, as this study progressed the researcher had collected at least one hundred folk terms, which could have been included terms. These were constantly checked with informants until six (status, hierarchy, machoness, non-femaleness, vulnerability, and institutions) were chosen to form the six domains of maleness. These six included terms were seen to cover a broadly theoretical interest, while at the same time allowing the researcher to be concerned with achieving depth to his study. The third component of the domain is the semantic relationship. For the relationship of one term to another to be valid, a semantic relationship needs to be established. In this instance, *Figure 12.2* shows the semantic relationship of the included terms of the domain maleness.

The analysis of the cover term, maleness, required the identification of relevant included terms, common ideas, and symbols used by the informants. This was done by observations, questioning informants, and interviews. The major symbols were determined through the use of common phrases and by implication and inference within the interview transcripts. The full taxonomy for the cover term, maleness, focusses on the six domains, but could have quite easily encompassed a great deal more.

Taxonomic analysis (Stage 8)

An understanding of the semantic relationship is essential for a complete taxonomic analysis (in-depth study of a domain). The purpose of taxonomic analysis is to develop a taxonomy of terms, associated with the cover term through semantic relationships. The domain, maleness, has six cover terms and each of these many included terms. These included terms represent cultural symbols that are organised through four (out of a possible nine) universal semantic relationships (*Figure 12.3*).

'Maleness is a way to do nursing' is the primary ethnographic theme of this thesis. Within the study focus of maleness, there are six central cover terms (strictly speaking, domains of maleness). Each of these have overlapping semantic relationships, which organise the cultural meaning of symbols referring to aspects of maleness. for example, the term, status, has the included terms: leadership, experience, authority, self-respect, confidence, doing the rough jobs, as just a few of its included terms. These included terms all have semantic relationship with the cover term 'status is a way to do maleness'. For example, leadership is a way to do status, authority is a result of status, and having self-respect is used to do status. These three different, semantic relationships were identified through informants being asked specific structural questions. The aim of the taxonomic analysis, in this study, was to enable the researcher to compile taxonomies of included terms of maleness, by nature of their semantic relationship. By doing this, the researcher was able to begin understanding how informants perceived maleness as having cultural meaning.

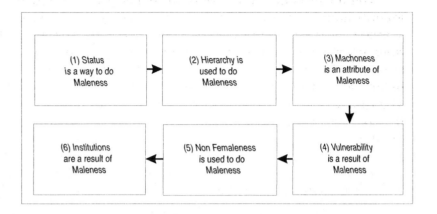

Figure 12.2 : The six ethnographic domains of maleness

● Strict inclusion	X is a kind of Y
● Spatial	X is a place in Y, X is a part of Y
● Cause-effect	X is a result of Y, X is a cause of Y
● Rationale	X is a reason for doing Y
● Location for action	X is a place for doing Y
● Function	X is used for Y
● Means-end	X is a way to do Y
● Sequence	X is a step (stage) in Y
● Attribution	X is an attribute (characteristic) of Y

Figure 12.3: The nine universal semantic relationships (Adapted from Spradley (1979: p11))

- *Domain*: the major symbolic category representing the overall idea addressed within the study—maleness
- *Included Term*: those terms directly related to the domain or to a sub-set of included terms
- *Cover Term*: the label given to any included term that is related to other included terms, through a semantic relationship.

Componential analysis (Stage 10)

The aim of componential analysis is to firm up the understanding of the relationship between included terms and the cover term. The basic idea is to use means that allow for included terms to be identified and then contrasted against other terms. The easiest way to perform this task is to ask contrast questions. As a method of analysis, componential analysis enabled the researcher to qualify the difference between included terms, such as authority and status in the first instance, and all the ways that male nurses are vulnerable towards the latter stages of data collection.

The DRS lends itself to the analysis and description of cultural symbols that are concrete, but it should be noted that one weakness of the DRS framework is its inability to provide a clear examination of more ambiguous symbols. The phrases and expressions given by the informants of the study, although recognisable, are not concrete. They constantly have double, or even more meanings. For example, the terms 'blagging' (bluffing your way through an interaction) and 'playing the fool' both have multiple meanings, upon which informants will not necessarily agree. Even in the best scientific endeavour, it is difficult to induce a universal meaning. Yet it is possible, by using the whole of the data', to ascertain 'the use' of these terms.

Post-structural analysis

The theme analysis (Stage 12) consolidated the six ethnographic domains shown in *Figure 12.2*. The taxonomies of included terms also allowed for the application of further theoretical exploration and analysis. This was achieved by applying a number of post-structural theoretical positions to the ethnographic themes. This progression allowed itself easily, due to the same epistemological foundations. Applying post-structural theory meant thinking about all events, meanings, observations, and the like, as clusters of signs and symbols, which must follow the same semiotic principles and have a similar functioning structure (e.g. signifier + signified = sign) to produce meaning that is not necessarily transposed via the spoken word.

The analysis (Phase two), which took two years, made use of a number of primary post-structural themes. These are now listed with their principle theorist:

- Myths (Barthes, 1996): the analysis of ideological connotations in culture using an extension of Saussurean semiotic discipline, e.g. the ethnographic theme of hierarchy can be seen to hide many connotations related to male nurses needing to exert power, 'climb to the top', and so on. *A questioning and interrogating of 'meaning'*

- Discourse (Foucault, 1980): an analysis that attempts to locate the nature of subjectivization of subject *identity* by discourse (powerful ideological structures), and explain how power and knowledge maintains particular cultural resonance. *A questioning of Identity*

- Simulation (Baudrillard, 1994): an analysis of reality, truth, and authenticity. The way that cultural signs and symbols are self-referential and refer to themselves, and cannot always be trusted to give a true meaning about cultural reality. *A questioning of reality, truth and authenticity*

- Deconstruction (Derrida, 1976): analysing the metaphysical reliance placed on meaning. *A questioning of meaning*

- Narratives (Lyotard, 1979): analysing the grand narratives that are seen to provide conceptual wholes to reality. *A questioning of meaning and reality.*

It can be seen that, by applying post-structural theory, the researcher has been able to extend the originality of his research and acknowledge that the present day theory has to rely upon an evolution of theoretical assumptions. The methodologically structured use of the DRS, combined with the more radical application of post-structural thought, provided a more complete and questioning study and thesis development.

The DRS is suited to the study of social structures and was flexible enough to allow the guiding question: 'What is happening here?' and then advance more questions using the initial data collected. The data was carefully analysed in an on-going manner in parallel with data collection. This gave the researcher the flexibility with informants, and allowed him the luxury of an immediacy; that is, a feeling that he was in immediate/close touch with his enquiry and his informants. Likewise, the development of domains, taxonomies, and a specific framework of analysis enabled the data sought to reflect the data collected. Hence, the progressive and developmental emphasis within the overall research sequence.

References

Aamodt A (1982) Examining ethnography for nurse researchers. *West J Nurs Res* **4**(2): 209–21

Agar MH (1976) 'Themes Revisited: Some Problems in Cognitive Anthropology '. Unpublished paper, Department of Anthropology, University of Houston.

Agar MH (1986) *Speaking of Ethnography*. Sage, Newbury Park, CA

Andersen ML, Collins PH (1992) Preface. In: Andersen ML, Collins PH (eds). *Race, Class and Gender*. Wadsworth, Belmont, CA

Austin R (1977) Sex and gender in the future of nursing, I. *Nurs Times* **73**(34): 113–16

Barthes R (1996) *Mythologies*. (Trans. Annette Lavers).Vintage Press, London

Basso K (1972) Ice travel among the fourth Norman slave: Folk taxonomies and cultural rules. *Language Society* **1**: 31–49

Batey MV, Lewis FM (1982) Clarifying autonomy and accountability in nursing service. *J Nurs Admin* **12**(9): 13–18

Baudrillard J (1994) *Simulacre and Simulation*. University of Michigan, Michigan

Bem S (1974) The measurement of psychological androgyny. *J Consult Clin Psychol* **42**: 155–62

Bloor M (1978) On the analysis of observational data: A discussion of the worth and uses of inductive techniques and respondent validation. *Sociology* **12**(3): 545–57

Bly R (1992) *Iron John: A Book about Men*. Element Press, Shaftesbury, Dorset and Rockport, Mass

Bogdan R, Taylor S (1975) *Introduction to Qualitative Research Methods: A Phenomenological Approach to the Social Sciences*. Wiley, New York

Boston Medical and Surgical Journal (1896) **136**: 214

Bowlby J (1969) *Attachment and Loss, Vol I: Attachment*. Basic Books, New York.

Bowlby J (1973) *Attachment and Loss, Vol I: Separation, Anxiety and Anger*. Basic Books, New York.

Bowlby J (1979) *The Making and Breaking of Affectional Bonds*. Tavistock, London

Bowman GS, Thompson DR (1995) Strategies for organising care. In: Schober JE, Hinchliff SM, eds. *Towards Advancing Nursing Practice*. Arnold Press, London: 222

Brink P (1976) *Transcultural Nursing: A Book of Readings*. Waveland Press Inc, Illinois

Brouse S (1995) The Theoretical Framework. In: Talbot L, ed. *Principles and Practice of Nursing Research* Mosby, St Louis: 141–67

Brown RGS, Stones RWH (1972) Personality and intelligence characterisitics of male nurses. *Int J Nurs Stud* **9**: 167–77

Buchbinder D (1998) *Performance Anxieties: Re-producing Masculinity*. Allen & Unwin, St Leonards, Australia

Burns RB (1977) Male and female perceptions of their own and other sex. *Br J Social Clin Psychol* **16**: 213–300

Butler J (1990) *Gender Trouble: From Parody to Politics, Feminism and the Subversion of Identity*. Routledge, New York

Byerly E (1969) The nurse researcher as participant observer in a nursing setting. *Nurs Res* **18**(3): 230–36

Cameron D (1985) *Feminism and Linguistic Theory*. Macmillan, London

Campbell M (1984) Information Systems and Management of Hospital Nursing: A Study in Social Organization of Knowledge. University of Toronto, Ontario

Carli L (1997) Biology does not create gender differences in personality. In: Walsh M, ed. *Women, Men and Gender: Ongoing Debates*. Yale University Press, New Haven: 44–57

Carr G (1996) Themes relating to sexuality that emerged from a discourse analysis of the Nursing Times during 1980–1990. *J Adv Nurs* **24**: 196–212

Chodorow N (1978) *The Reproduction of Mothering*. University of California Press, Berkley, CA

Conklin H (1962) Lexicographical treatment of folk taxonomies. In: Householder F, Sapoota, S, eds. *Problems of Lexicography* Indiana University Research Center in Anthropology, Folklore and Linguistics: Publication 21: 119–41

Connell RW (1987) *Gender and Power*. Polity Press, New York

Connell RW (1995) *Masculinities*. Polity Press, New York

Crowe M (1998) The power of the word: some post -structural considerations of qualitative approaches in nursing research. *J Adv Nurs* **28**(2): 339–44

Davies C (1995) *Gender and the Professional Predicament in Nursing*. Open University Press, Buckingham

de Beauvoir S (1949) The Second Sex. Originally published in English (1953) by Jonathan Cape Ltd, London

Delmar R (1986) What is feminism? In: Mitchel J, Oakly A (eds), *What Is Feminism?* Basil Blackwell, London

de Montigny G (1995) *Social Working: An Ethnography of Front Line Practice*. University of Toronto Press, Toronto

Denzin NK (1997) *Interpretive Ethnography: Ethnographic Practices for the 21st Century*. Sage, Califomia.

Derrida J (1976) *Of Grammatology*. Johns Hopkins University Press, London/Baltimore

Dickson GL (1995) Philosophical orientation of qualitative research. In: Talbot LA, ed. *Principles and Practice of Nursing Research*. Mosby Year Book, St Louis

Dingwall R (1972) Nursing: towards a male dominated occupation? *Nurs Times* **68**: 1294–95

References

Dingwall R (1980) Ethics and ethnography. *Sociolog Rev* **28**(4): 871–91

Douglas J (1970) *Understanding Everyday Life: Toward the Reconstruction of Sociological Knowledge*. Aldine Publishing Company, Chicago

du Gay P, ed (1997) *Production of Culture/Cultures of Production*. Sage Publications, London

Durkheim E (1967) *The Division of Labour in Society*. The Free Press, New York

Eagly A (1995) Transforming the debate on sexual inequality: From biological difference to institutionalized androcentrism. In: Chrisler C, Golden C, Rozee P, eds. *Lectures on the Psychology of Women*. McGraw-Hill, New York

Erikson E (1963) Childhood and Society. W W Norton Publishing, London

Evans M, Litowitz B, Markowitz J, Smith R, Werner O (1977) Lexical/semantic relations: A comparative survey. Unpublished manuscript. Department of Anthropology, Macalester College, St. Paul, Minn

Faith K (1994) Resistance: Lessons from Foucault and feminism. In: Radtke H, Starn H, eds. *Power/Gender*. Sage Publications, London: 36–66

Fawcett J (1994) *Analysis and Evaluation of Conceptual Models of Nursing*, 3rd edn. Davis Publications, Philadelphia

Field P, Morse J (1991) *Nursing Research: The Application of Qualitative Approaches*. Chapman and Hall, London

Fine M, Gordon S (1989) Feminist transformations of/despite psychology. In: Crawford M, Gentry M, eds. *Gender and Thought*. Springer-Verlag, New York: 146–74

Firestone S (1972) *The Dialectic of Sex*. Paladin Press, London

Fliegel ZO (1986) Women's development in analytic theory. In: Alpert JL, ed. *Psychoanalysis and Women: Contemporary Reappraisals*. The Analytic Press, Hillsdale, NJ: 3–31

Foucault M (1971) *Madness and Civilization*. Tavistock Press, London

Foucault M (1973) *The Order of Things: An Archaeology of the Human Sciences*. (Trans. non-listed). Random House Vintage Books, New York

Foucault M (1980) *Power/knowledge. Selected Interviews and Other Writings 1972-1977*. Harvester Press, Brighton

Freilich M (1970) *Marginal Natives: Anthropologists at Work*. Harper and Row, New York

Freud S (1995) *The Complete Works of Sigmund Freud*. (Strachey J, ed) Hogarth Press, London

Freud S (1997) The Interpretation of Dreams (Brill AA, trans) Wordsworth Classics, Hertfordshire

Game A, Pringle R (1983) *Gender at Work*. Pluto Press, London

Garfinkel H (1967) *Studies in Ethnomethodology*. Prentice Hall, New Jersey

Gilmore D (1990) *Manhood in the Making: Cultural Concepts of Masculinity*. Yale University Press, New Haven

Glaser B (1978) *Theoretical Sensitivity*. The Sociology Press, San Francisco

Glaser B, Strauss A (1967) *The Discovery of Grounder Theory: Strategies for Qualitative Research*. Aldine Publishers, Chicago

Goetz J, Lecompte M (1984) *Ethnography and Qualitative Design in Educational Research*. Academic Press, Orlando

Goffman E (1959) *The Presentation of Self in Everyday Life*. Anchor Books, New York (Pelican Books, Middlesex, (1969))

Goffman E (1961) *Asylums*. Anchor Books, Doubleday & Co, New York. (Pelican Books, Middlesex (1968))

Goodenough W (1957) Cultural anthropology and linguistics. In: Garvin P, ed. *Report of the Seventh Annual Round Table Meeting on Linguistics and Language Study*. Georgetown University Monograph Series on Language and Linguistics: 9. Georgetown University, Washington DC

Gorman C (1992) Sizing up the Sexes. *Time* **Jan 20**: 42–51

Gould SJ (1981) *The Mismeasure of Man*. Norton, New York

Greer G (1971) *The Female Eunuch*. Paladin, London

Greer G (1984) *Sex and Destiny: The Politics of Human Fertility*. Martin Secker & Warburg, London

Greer G (1999) *The Whole Woman*. Anchor, London

Gregor F (1994) *The Social Organization of Knowledge in the Educative Work of Nursing*. Dalhousie University, Halifax

Gubrium J (1988) *Analysing Field Reality*. Qualitative Research Methods Series No 8. Sage, Newbury Park

Gubrium J, Buckholdt D (1982) *Describing Care: Image and Practice in Rehabilitation*. Oelschlager, Gunn and Rain, Cambridge: Mass

Gubrium J, Holstein J (1987) The private image: experimental location and method in family studies. *J Marriage Fam* **49**: 773–86

Hall S (1997) Introduction. In: Hall S, ed. *Representation. Cultural Representations and Signifying Practices*. Sage Publications, London: 1–13

Hall S, du Gay P, eds (1996) *Questions of Cultural Identity*. Sage Publications, London

Hammersley M (1992) *What's Wrong With Ethnography: Methodological Explorations*. Routledge, London

Hansen J (1976) Ethnography of Second Grade Boys Playing Matchbox Cars. Unpublished seminar paper, Department of Anthropology. Malcalester College, St. Paul, Minn

Haralambos M, Holborn M (1995) *Sociology: Themes and Perspectives*, 4th edn. Collins Educational Publishers, London

Hartsock N (1990) Foucault on power: a theory for women? In: Nicholson L, ed. *Feminism and Postmodernism*. Routledge, London: 157–75

Hawkes T (1977) *Structuralism and Semiotics*. Methuen, London

Henderson A (1994) Power and knowledge in nursing practice: The contribution of Foucault. *J Adv Nurs* **20**: 935–39

Heritage J (1984) *Garfinkel and Ethnomethodology*. Polity Press, Cambridge

Hesselbart S (1977) Women doctors win and male nurses lose: a study of sex role and occupational stereotypes. *Sociol Work Occup* **4**(1): 49

Hewison A (1995) Nurses' power in interactions with patients. *J Adv Nurs* **21**: 75–82

Hewitt R (1997) 'Boxed-out' and 'Taxing'. In: Johnson S, Meinhof UH, eds. *Language and Masculinity*. Blackwell Publishers, Oxford: 27–46

Hicks C (1996) The potential impact of gender stereotypes for nursing research. *J Adv Nurs* **24**: 1006–13

Hite S (1987) *The Hite Report on Love, Passion and Emotional Violence*. Alfred A Knopf, New York

Hite S (1994) *The Hite Report on the Family—Growing Up under Patriarchy*. Bloomsbury Publishing, London

Hoffman H (1970) Notes on the personality traits of student nurses. *Psycholog Rep* **27**: 1004

Holland C (1993) An ethnographic study of nursing culture as an exploration for determining the existence of a system of ritual. *J Adv Nurs* **18**: 1461–70

Hollway W, Jefferson T (1996) PC or Not PC : Sexual harassment and the question of ambivalence. *J Hum Relations* **49**(3): 373–93

Holyoake D (1999) Who's the boss?: Children 's perception of hospital hierarchy. *Paediatr Nurs* **11**(5): 33–36

Huntington A (1996) Nursing research reframed by the inescapable reality of practice: A personal encounter. *Nurs Inq* **3**: 167–71

Hyde J (1985) *Half the Human Experience*, 3rd edn. Heath, Lexington, Mass, DC

Irigaray L (1992) *Culture of Difference*, (trans. Alison Martin). Routledge, New York

James N (1992) Care = organisation + physical labour + emotional labour. *Sociol Health Illness* **14**(4): 488–509

Jolley M (1989) The professionalisation of nursing: the uncertain path. In: Jolley M, Allen P, eds. *Current Issues in Nursing*. Chapman Hall, London

Kay M (1979) Disease concepts in Barrio today. In: Bately V, ed. *Communicating Nursing Research*. Boulder, California, Vol6, p 185-194.

Keddy B, Jones GM, Jacobs P, Burton H, Rogers M (1986) The doctor-nurse relationship: an historical perspective. *J Adv Nurs* **11**: 745–53

Kimball S, Watson J (1972) *Crossing Cultural Boundaries: The Anthropological Experience*. Chandler Publishers, Chicago

Kitzinger C (1987) *The Social Construction of Lesbianism*. Sage, London

Kock T (1994) Establishing rigour in qualitative research: the decision trail. *J Adv Nurs* **19**: 976–86

Kristeva J (1982) *Powers of Horror. An Essay on Abjection*, (trans. Leon Roudiez). Columbia University Press, New York.

Kroeber A, Kluckhohn C (1952) *Culture: A Critical Review of Concepts and Definitions*, Vol XLVII, No 1. Papers of the Peabody Museum of American Archaeology and Ethnology. Harvard University, Cambridge

Kuzel A (1992) Sampling in qualitative inquiry. In: Crabtree B, Miller W, eds. *Doing Qualitative Research*. Sage, Newbury Park

Lacan J (1968) *The Language of the Self*, (Wilden A, trans and ed). Johns Hopkins University Press, Baltimore

Laing R, Esterson A (1964) *Sanity, Madness and the Family*. Tavistock Publication, London

Lemkau JP (1984) Men in female-dominated professions: distinguishing personality and background features. *J Vocat Behav* 24: 110

Lincoln YS, Guba EG (1985) *Naturalistic-Inquiry*. Sage, Beverly Hills, CA

Lincoln YS, Guba EG (1989) *Fourth Generation Evaluation*. Sage Publications, California

Lott B (1990) Dual natures or learned behaviour: the challenge to feminist psychology. In: Hare-Mustin R, Marecek J, eds. *Making a Difference: Psychology and the Construction of Gender*. Yale University Press, New Haven: 65–101

Lukes S (1974) *Power: A Radical View*. Macmillan Press, London

Lynn BN, Vaden AG, Vaden RE (1975) The challenges of men in a woman's world. *Pub Personnel Man* 4(1): 4–17

Lyotard J (1979) *The Postmodern Condition*, trans. Geoffrey Bennington and Brian Massuni. Minnesota University Press, Minneapolis

Mac an Ghaill M (1985) *The Making of Men: Masculinities, Sexualities and Schooling*. Open University Press, Milton Keynes

Maccoby E, Jacklin C (1974) *The Psychology of Sex Differences*. Stanford University Press, Stanford, CA

Malinowski B (1954, originally published in 1922) *Argonauts of the Western Pacific*. Routledge & Kegan Paul, London

Manicom A (1988) Constituting Class Relations: The Social Organization of Teachers' Work. Unpublished doctoral thesis. Ontario Institute of Education, Toronto

Mariano C (1995) The Qualitative Research Process. In: Talbot L, ed. *Principles and Practice of Nursing Research*. Mosby, St Louis: 463–91

Marshall C, Rossman G (1989) *Designing Qualitative Research*. Sage Publications, London

Matlin M (1996) *The Psychology of Women*, 3rd edn. Harcourt Brace, Fort Worth, Texas

Mead GH (1962) *Mind; Self and Society*. University of Chicago Press, Chicago

Mednick M (1989) On the politics of psychological constructs: stop the band-wagon, I want to get off. *Am Psychol* 44: 1118–23

Merriam S (1988) *Case Study Research in Education: A Qualitative Approach*. Jossey-Bass, San Francisco

Millett K (1970) *Sexual Politics*. Doubleday Press, New York

Mitchell J (1971) *Women's Estate*. Penguin, London

Moir A, Moir B (1999) *Why Men Don't Iron: The New reality of Gender Differences*. Harper Collins Publishers, Hammersmith, London

Molm LD (1986) Gender, power and legitimation: a test of three theories. *Am J Sociol* 91(6): 1356–86

Morton T (1997) *Altered Mates: The Man Question*. Allen & Unwin, St Leonards, Australia

Naish J (1995) Give up your power. *Nurs Man* 2(6): 6–7

Nash J (1976) The short and long of it: legitimizing motives for running. In: Nash J, Spradley J, eds. *Sociology: A Descriptive Approach.* Rand McNally, Chicago: 161–81

Nash J (1977) Decoding the runner's wardrobe. In: *Conformity and Conflict: Readings in Cultural Anthropology,* 3rd edn. Little Brown Publishing, Boston: 172–86

Nash J, McCurdy D (1989) Cultural knowledge and systems of knowing. *Sociolog Enq* **59**(2): 117–26

Ng R (1984) Immigrant Women and the State: A Study of the Social Organization of Knowledge. Unpublished doctoral thesis, Ontario Institute of Education, Toronto

Nixon S (1997) Exhibiting Masculinity. In: Hall S, ed. *Representation: Cultural Representations and Signifying Practices.* Sage Publications, London: 291–338

Nuttall P (1983) Male takeover or female giveaway? *Nurs Times* **79**(2): 10–11

O'Donnell M (1997) *Introduction to Sociology,* 4th edn. Thomas Nelson and Sons, Surrey

Ohlen I, Segesten K (1998) The professional identity of the nurse: concept analysis and development. *J Adv Nurs* **28**(4): 720–27

Orem D (1991) *Nursing Concepts of Practice,* 4th edn. Mosby Year Book, St Louis

Paglia C (1992) *Sexual Personae: Art and Decadence from Nefertiti to Emily Dickinson.* Penguin, London

Parfitt B (1996) Using Spradley: an ethnosemantic approach to research. *J Adv Nurs* **24**: 341–49

Parse R (1981) *Man-Living-Health: A Theory of Nursing.* John Wiley, New York

Parse R (1992) Human becoming: Parse's theory of nursing. *Nurs Sci Q* **5**(1): 35–42

Parsons T (1951) *The Social System.* Routledge, London & New York

Pateman C (1988) *The Sexual Contract.* Polity Press, Cambridge

Patton MQ (1990) *Qualitative Evaluation and Research Methods,* 2nd edn. Sage, Newbury Park, CA

Peplau H (1988) *Interpersonal Relations in Nursing,* 2nd edn. Macmillan, London

Phoca S, Wright R (1999) *Introducing Post-feminism.* Icon Books, Cambridge, UK

Pierce C (1931) *Collected Papers.* Harvard University Press, Cambridge

Pleck JH, Sawyer J (1974) *Men and Masculinity.* Prentice Hall, Englewood Cliffs, NJ

Pontin DJT (1988) The use of profile similarity indices and the Bem sex role inventory in determining the sex role characterization of a group of male and female nurses. *J Adv Nurs* **13**: 768–74

Poster M (1984) *Foucault, Marxism and History.* Polity Press, Cambridge

Ragucci A (1972) The ethnographic approach and nursing research. *Nurs Res* **21**: 485–90

Ratcliffe P (1996) Gender differences in career progress in nursing: towards a non-essentialist structural theory. *J Adv Nurs* **23**: 389–95

Robinson K (1992) The nursing workforce: aspects of inequality. In: Robinson I, Gray A, Elkan R, eds. *Policy Issues in Nursing*. Open University Press, Milton Keynes: 24–37

Rogers M (1970) *An Introduction to the Theoretical Basis of Nursing*. PA Davis, Philadelphia

Royal College of Nursing (1985) *Commission on Nursing Education. The Education of Nurses: A New Dispensation*. Royal College of Nursing, London

Rutty J (1998) The nature of philosophy of science, theory and knowledge relating to nursing and professionalism. *J Adv Nurs* **28**(2): 243–50

Sacks H (1992) Jefferson G, ed, *Lectures on Conversation*, Vol 1 and 2. Basil Blackwell, Oxford

Saussure P (1959) *Course in General Linguistics*, trans by W Baskin . Philosophical Library Press, New York

Scott S, Morgan D (1993) *Essays on the Sociology of the Body*. The Palmer Press, London

Shapiro L (1990) 'Guns and Dolls '. *Newsweek* **May 28**: 56–65

Sharpe S (1972) *Recreating Sexual Politics*, 2nd edn.. Penguin, Harmondsworth

Silverman D (1993) *Interpreting Qualitative Data: Methods for Analysing Talk, Text and Interaction*. Sage Publications, London

Sines D (1994) The arrogance of power : a reflection on contemporary mental health nursing practice. *J Adv Nurs* **20**: 894–903

Smith P (1993) Nursing as an occupation. In: Taylor S, Field D, eds. *Sociology of Health and Health Care*. Blackwell Science, Oxford: 205–23

Spelman EV (1988) *Inessential Woman: Problems of Exclusion in Feminist Thought*. Beacon Press, Boston

Spindler G (1970) *Being an Anthropologist*. Holt, Rinehart and Winston, New York

Spradley J (1970) *You Owe Yourself a Drink: An Ethnography of Urban Nomads*. Little, Brown & Co, Boston

Spradley J (1979) *The Ethnographic Interview*. Holt, Rinehart and Winston, New York

Spradley J (1980) *Participant Observation*. Holt, Rinehart and Winston, New York

Spradley J, McCurdy D (1975) *Anthropology: The Cultural Perspective*. Wiley, New York

Strauss CL (1963) *Structural Anthropology*, trans by C Jacobsen and BG Schoepf. University of Chicago Press, Chicago

Strauss CL (1963a) *Totemism Today*, trans by R Needharn. Beacon Press, Boston

Strauss CL (1966) *The Savage Mind*, trans by G Weidenfeld and Nicolson Ltd. University of Chicago Press, Chicago

Strauss A, Corbin J (1990) *Basic of Qualitative Research: Grounded Theory Procedures and Techniques*. Sage, Newbury Park, CA

Talbot L (1995) Populations and samples. In: Talbot L, ed. *Principles and Practice of Nursing Research*. Mosby, St Louis: 240–62

Tesch R (1990) *Qualitative Research: Analysis Types and Software Tools*. The Palmer Press, Bristol

Thwaites T, Davis L, Mules W (1994) *Tools for Cultural Studies: An Introduction*. Macmillan, South Melbourne

Thomas D (1993) *Not Guilty: In Defence of the Modern Man*. Weidenfeld and Nicolson, London

Tolson A (1977) *The Limits of Masculinity*. Tavistock Publications, London

Touhey JC (1974) Effects of additional women professionals on ratings of occupational prestige and desirability. *J App Social Psychol* **29**: 86

Townsend E (1996) Institutional ethnography: A method for showing how the context shapes practice. *Occ Ther J Res* **16**(3): 179–99

Tuck I (1995) Qualitative designs. In: Talbot L, ed. *Principles and Practice of Nursing Research*. Mosby, St Louis: 437–62

Unger R (1989) Sex, gender and epistemology. In: Crawford M, Gentry M eds. *Gender and Thought*. Springer-Verlag, New York

Unger R (1992) Will the real sex difference please stand up? *Fem Psychol* **2**(2): 231–8

Unger R, Crawford M (1992) *Women and Gender: A Feminist Psychology*. Temple University Press, Philadelphia

Walsh MR (1977) *Doctors Wanted: No Women Need Apply*. Yale University Press, New Haven

Walsh MR, ed (1997) *Women, Men, and Gender*. Yale University Press, New Jersey

Watson C (1997) Gender versus power as a predictor of negotiation. In: Walsh M, ed. *Women, Men and Gender: Ongoing Debates*. Yale University Press, New Haven: 145–54

Weber M (1947) *The Theory of Social and Economic Organisations*, trans. Henderson AM, Parsons T; revised and edited by Parsons T). Oxford University Press, Oxford (First published in German in 1922)

Weeks J (1981) *Sex, Politics and Society*. Longman, Harlow

Weeks J (1985) *Sexuality and its Discontents*. Routledge, London

Werner O, Schoepfle G (1987) *Systematic Field-work*, Vol 1–2). Sage, Newbury Park

Wilson H (1985) *Research in Nursing*. Addison-Wesley, Menlo Park, CA

Wrong DH (1979) *Power: Its Forms, Bases and Uses*. Basil Blackwell, Oxford

Index